T0348624

Device-Associated Infections

Editor

VIVIAN H. CHU

INFECTIOUS DISEASE CLINICS OF NORTH AMERICA

www.id.theclinics.com

Consulting Editor
HELEN W. BOUCHER

December 2018 • Volume 32 • Number 4

ELSEVIER

1600 John F. Kennedy Boulevard • Suite 1800 • Philadelphia, Pennsylvania, 19103-2899.
http://www.theclinics.com

INFECTIOUS DISEASE CLINICS OF NORTH AMERICA Volume 32, Number 4
December 2018 ISSN 0891–5520, ISBN-13: 978-0-323-64330-6

Editor: Kerry Holland
Developmental Editor: Donald Mumford

Infectious Disease Clinics of North America (ISSN 0891–5520) is published in March, June, September, and December by Elsevier Inc., 360 Park Avenue South, New York, NY 10010-1710. Periodicals postage paid at New York, NY and additional mailing offices. Subscription prices are $319.00 per year for US individuals, $629.00 per year for US institutions, $100.00 per year for US students, $379.00 per year for Canadian individuals, $785.00 per year for Canadian institutions, $428.00 per year for international individuals, $785.00 per year for international institutions, and $200.00 per year for Canadian and international students. To receive student rate, orders must be accompanied by name of affiliated institution, date of term, and the *signature* of program/residency coordinator on institution letterhead. Orders will be billed at individual rate until proof of status is received. Foreign air speed delivery is included in all *Clinics* subscription prices. All prices are subject to change without notice. **POSTMASTER**: Send address changes to *Infectious Disease Clinics of North America*, Elsevier Health Sciences Division, Subcription Customer Service, 3251 Riverport Lane, Maryland Heights, MO 63043. **Customer Service: 1-800-654-2452 (US). From outside of the US and Canada, call 1-314-447-8871. Fax: 1-314-447-8029. E-mail: JournalsCustomerService-usa@elsevier.com (print support) or JournalsOnlineSupport-usa@elsevier.com (online support).**

Infectious Disease Clinics of North America is also published in Spanish by Editorial Inter-Médica, Junin 917, 1er A 1113, Buenos Aires, Argentina.

Reprints. For copies of 100 or more, of articles in this publication, please contact the Commercial Reprints Department, Elsevier Inc., 360 Park Avenue South, New York, New York 10010-1710. Tel. 212-633-3874, Fax: 212-633-3820, E-mail: reprints@elsevier.com.

Infectious Disease Clinics of North America is covered in *MEDLINE/PubMed (Index Medicus), Current Contents/Clinical Medicine, Science Citation Alert, SCISEARCH,* and *Research Alert.*

Contributors

CONSULTING EDITOR

HELEN W. BOUCHER, MD, FIDSA, FACP
Director, Infectious Diseases Fellowship Program, Division of Geographic Medicine and Infectious Diseases, Tufts Medical Center, Associate Professor of Medicine, Tufts University School of Medicine, Boston, Massachusetts, USA

EDITOR

VIVIAN H. CHU, MD, MHS
Associate Professor, Division of Infectious Diseases, Duke University School of Medicine, Durham, North Carolina, USA

AUTHORS

CHRISTOPHER J. ARNOLD, MD
Assistant Professor, Division of Infectious Diseases and International Health, University of Virginia Health System, Charlottesville, Virginia, USA

ELENA BEAM, MD
Assistant Professor of Medicine, Division of Infectious Disease, Department of Internal Medicine, Mayo Clinic, Rochester, Minnesota, USA

CAROL E. CHENOWETH, MD
Department of Internal Medicine and Antimicrobial Stewardship Program, Michigan Medicine, Ann Arbor, Michigan, USA

VIVIAN H. CHU, MD, MHS
Associate Professor, Division of Infectious Diseases, Duke University School of Medicine, Durham, North Carolina, USA

AMAL GHARAMTI, MD
Division of Infectious Diseases, Department of Internal Medicine, American University of Beirut, Beirut, Lebanon

JONATHAN D. GREIN, MD
Department of Hospital Epidemiology, Division of Infectious Diseases, Cedars-Sinai Medical Center, Associate Clinical Professor, David Geffen School of Medicine at UCLA, Los Angeles, California, USA

MARGARET M. HANNAN, MD
Department of Clinical Microbiology, Mater Misericordiae University Hospital, University College Dublin, Dublin, Ireland

ZEINA A. KANAFANI, MD, MS, CIC
Division of Infectious Diseases, Department of Internal Medicine, American University of Beirut, Associate Professor of Medicine, American University of Beirut Medical Center, Beirut, Lebanon

RAJENDRA KARNATAK, MBBS
Postdoctoral Fellow, Division of Infectious Diseases, University of Nebraska Medical Center, Omaha, Nebraska, USA

TAHANIYAT LALANI, MBBS, MHS
Associate Professor, Preventive Medicine and Biostatistics, Uniformed Services University of the Health Sciences, Bethesda, Maryland, USA

SARAH S. LEWIS, MD, MPH
Division of Infectious Diseases, Department of Medicine, Duke University School of Medicine, Duke University Medical Center, Duke Center for Antimicrobial Stewardship and Infection Prevention, Durham, North Carolina, USA

REKHA K. MURTHY, MD, FRCPC
Professor of Medicine, Division of Infectious Diseases, Associate Chief Medical Officer, Department of Medical Affairs, Cedars-Sinai Medical Center, Professor of Clinical Medicine, David Geffen School of Medicine at UCLA, Los Angeles, California, USA

DOUGLAS OSMON, MD
Professor of Medicine, Division of Infectious Disease, Departments of Medicine and Orthopedic Surgery, Mayo Clinic, Rochester, Minnesota, USA

ROBIN PATEL, MD
Professor of Microbiology, Professor of Medicine, Elizabeth P. and Robert E. Allen Professor of Individualized Medicine, Divisions of Clinical Microbiology and Infectious Diseases, Departments of Laboratory Medicine and Pathology and Medicine, Mayo Clinic, Rochester, Minnesota, USA

MARK E. RUPP, MD
Professor and Chief, Division of Infectious Diseases, University of Nebraska Medical Center, Omaha, Nebraska, USA

JESSICA SEIDELMAN, MD
Division of Infectious Diseases, Department of Medicine, Duke University School of Medicine, Duke University Medical Center, Duke Center for Antimicrobial Stewardship and Infection Prevention, Durham, North Carolina, USA

EMILY K. SHUMAN, MD
Departments of Internal Medicine and Infection Prevention and Epidemiology, Michigan Medicine, Ann Arbor, Michigan, USA

TEE K. TEOH, MD
Department of Clinical Microbiology, Mater Misericordiae University Hospital, University College Dublin, Dublin, Ireland

YU MI WI, MD, PhD
Division of Infectious Diseases, Department of Internal Medicine, Samsung Changwon Hospital, Sungkyunkwan University, Changwon-si, Gyeongsangnam-do, Korea

Contents

Despite recent gains, intravascular catheter–related bloodstream infection (CRBSI) remains an important clinical problem resulting in significant morbidity, mortality, and excess economic cost. Successful prevention of CRBSI requires careful attention to insertion and maintenance protocols as well as judicious application of innovative technologic advancements. Appropriate treatment of CRBSI depends on a well-considered diagnosis, correct antimicrobial choice, removal of the offending device in many circumstances, and careful patient selection and application of antimicrobial lock therapy in patients in whom catheter salvage is attempted.

Vascular graft infection is a devastating complication of vascular reconstructive surgery. The infection can occur early in the postoperative period and is largely due to intraoperative contamination or by contiguous extension from a nearby infection. It can also occur years after implantation. Staphylococci remain the most common organisms and biofilm production makes eradication difficult. Factors commonly reported to predispose to vascular graft infection are periodontal disease, nasal colonization with *Staphylococcus aureus*, bacteremia, certain graft characteristics, diabetes mellitus, postoperative hyperglycemia, location of the incision, wound infection, and emergency procedure. Management consists of antibiotic and surgical therapy. Preventive methods are described.

Infections associated with cardiac implantable electronic devices are increasing and are associated with significant morbidity and mortality. This article reviews the epidemiology, microbiology, and risk factors for acquisition of these infections. The complex diagnostic and management strategies associated with these serious infections are reviewed with an emphasis on recent updates and advances, as well as existing controversies. Additionally, the latest in preventative strategies are reviewed.

Heart transplant remain the definitive therapy for end-stage heart failure but is limited by the availability of suitable donors. Ventricular assist devices (VAD) are designed as mechanical pumps to supplement or replace the function of damaged ventricles and maintain appropriate blood flow in patients with end-stage heart failure. Survival rates continue to increase in patient with VAD but infection remains a major cause of morbidity and mortality in VAD patients. The authors describe the current concepts regarding definitions, diagnosis, microbiology and principles of management in VAD-associated infections. The authors have also summarised the prevention strategies for infections in VAD patients.

Prosthetic joint infection occurs in a minority of arthroplasties performed; however, it brings a large burden to both the individual and society in terms of morbidity, mortality, and health care expenditure. Although prevention of prosthetic joint infection is becoming more effective, the number of total arthroplasties in patients with increasing comorbidities continues to rise, and the total number of diagnosed and managed prosthetic joint infections is expected to rise accordingly. Management is complex and involves a multispecialty approach.

In this review article, we discuss the epidemiology, microbiology, diagnosis, treatment and prevention of infections associated with cerebrospinal fluid shunts, cerebrospinal fluid drains, and deep brain stimulators. We also briefly discuss prevention strategies with appropriate antibiotics, devices, and operating room practices to decrease the risk of these infections.

Prosthetic breast implantation is a common surgical procedure for augmentation and reconstruction after mastectomy. The incidence of implant infection is 1% to 2.5% and is higher for reconstruction following mastectomy compared with augmentation. Most infections are caused by gram-positive pathogens, such as coagulase-negative staphylococci, Cutibacterium species, *Staphylococcus aureus*, and streptococci. Acute infections are usually associated with fever and breast pain, erythema, and drainage. Subacute infections may present with chronic pain, persistent drainage, failed healing of the incision site, or migration of the implant. Depending on severity of infection, patients are started on empiric intravenous or oral antibiotics and closely monitored.

Catheter-associated urinary tract infection remains one of the most prevalent, yet preventable, health care-associated infections. General prevention strategies include strict adherence to hand hygiene and antimicrobial stewardship. Duration of urinary catheterization is the most important modifiable risk factor. Targeted prevention strategies include limiting urinary catheter use; physician reminder systems, nurse-initiated discontinuation protocols, and automatic stop orders have successfully decreased catheter duration. Alternatives should be considered. If catheterization is necessary, proper aseptic practices for insertion and maintenance and closed catheter collection systems are essential for prevention. The use of bladder bundles and collaboratives aids in the effective implementation of prevention measures.

Gastrointestinal endoscopes are used for diagnostic and therapeutic purposes and are the most common medical device implicated in health care-associated outbreaks. Infections can be divided into endogenous or exogenous. Exogenous infections were associated with lapses in reprocessing. Recent outbreaks have occurred despite compliance with reprocessing guidelines and highlight the challenges with clearance of all organisms from the duodenoscopes and the potential role of biofilms in hindering adequate reprocessing. This review provides an overview of recent developments and the current understanding of the key contributing factors related to gastrointestinal endoscope-related infections and current approaches to identify and prevent these complications.

Treatment of medical device-related infections is challenging and recurrence is common. The main reason for this is that microorganisms adhere to the surfaces of medical devices and enter into a biofilm state in which they display distinct growth rates, structural features, and protection from antimicrobial agents and host immune mechanisms compared with their planktonic counterparts. This article reviews how microorganisms form biofilms and the mechanisms of protection against antimicrobial agents and the host immune system provided by biofilms. Also discussed are innovative strategies for the diagnosis of biofilm-associated infection and novel approaches to treatment and prevention of medical device-associated infections.

INFECTIOUS DISEASE CLINICS
OF NORTH AMERICA

Preface

Device-Associated Infections

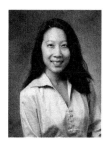

Vivian H. Chu, MD, MHS
Editor

Advances in health care have necessitated the use of devices, which are increasing in numbers and expanding in variety. In many cases, these devices are being used in increasingly older patients and in those with major comorbidities. For example, in a recent study of implantable cardioverter defibrillators, patients aged 70 to 79 accounted for 31% of implantations, while octogenarians accounted for 8% of implantations.[1] Ventricular assist devices (VAD), a life-saving therapy for patients with end-stage heart failure, are increasingly used as destination therapy (now nearly half of patients who receive a VAD).[2] The patients we treat are complex, and often the task of treating their device-related infections is not straightforward.

Biofilm formation is central to the theme of device-associated infections. It is because of the tenacity of biofilm that devices often need to be removed to provide the best chance for cure. In this issue, an article on biofilm focuses on this universal problem of medical devices and offers insights into the latest in biofilm research, such as antimicrobials that are able to penetrate biofilm and materials that inhibit biofilm formation.

Experts in the field have been chosen to summarize key features and to highlight recent advances in the prevention and management of important device-related infections. Some articles focus on common infections, such as intravascular catheter-related bloodstream infections, while others focus on highly specialized areas, such as VAD infections. Outbreaks of multidrug-resistant gram-negative infections related to gastrointestinal (GI) scopes received widespread attention recently and are relevant to all centers providing GI diagnostics. As such, an article on GI scope-related infections is included.

I hope that you will be fascinated by the scientific updates in this issue. How does shark skin inform the design of device surfaces? Is there a role for alpha-defensin in the diagnosis of prosthetic joint infections? Can antibacterial envelopes reduce the rate of infection in cardiovascular implantable electronic devices?

Infect Dis Clin N Am 32 (2018) ix–x
https://doi.org/10.1016/j.idc.2018.09.001
0891-5520/18/© 2018 Published by Elsevier Inc.

id.theclinics.com

While our authors have presented the newest and most interesting advances in the field, they have also reviewed the practicalities of managing these infections. Treating patients with device-related infections requires an individualized approach and careful consideration of antibiotics, device removal versus retention, and timing of device replacement, if applicable. Most of the time, with increasingly complex patients, these decisions are difficult to make.

Best of luck to those of you who are tackling these difficult decisions, and many thanks to our authors for creating this exceptional clinical resource.

Vivian H. Chu, MD, MHS
Division of Infectious Diseases
Duke University School of Medicine
Duke Box 102359
Durham, NC 27710, USA

E-mail address:
vivian.chu@duke.edu

REFERENCES

1. Yung D, Birnie D, Dorian P, et al. Survival after implantable cardioverter-defibrillator implantation in the elderly. Circulation 2013;127(24):2383–92.
2. Kirklin JK, Naftel DC, Pagani FD, et al. Seventh INTERMACS annual report: 15,000 patients and counting. J Heart Lung Transplant 2015;34(12):1495–504.

Intravascular Catheter–Related Bloodstream Infections

Mark E. Rupp, MD*, Rajendra Karnatak, MBBS

KEYWORDS

- Catheter-related bloodstream infection
- Central line–associated bloodstream infection • Central venous catheter
- Bacteremia • Health care–associated infection

KEY POINTS

- Approximately 30,000 to 40,000 episodes of catheter-related bloodstream infection (CRBSI) occur in the United States each year, resulting in a significantly increased odds of death and an estimated cost of $45,000 per event.
- Successful prevention of CRBSI requires application of practice-based measures, such as catheter insertion with the use of full sterile barrier precautions, checklists, and maintenance protocols, emphasizing sterile catheter access technique and catheter dressing integrity, as well as judicious application of evidence-based innovative technologic advances, such as antimicrobial-coated catheters, chlorhexidine-impregnated dressings, and passive port protectors.
- A diagnosis of CRBSI can often be made without catheter removal by application of the differential time to positivity blood culture assay.
- Increasing experience is being gained with successful catheter salvage and treatment without catheter removal using antimicrobial lock therapy.

BACKGROUND AND CLINICAL SIGNIFICANCE

Intravascular (IV) catheters, which include peripheral and midline venous catheters, subcutaneously tunneled and nontunneled central venous catheters (CVCs), peripherally inserted central catheters, totally indwelling devices (ie, ports), and arterial catheters (ACs) are essential and ubiquitous in health care. Although great strides have recently been achieved in the prevention of IV catheter–related infection, with an observed 50% reduction in central line–associated bloodstream infections (CLABSIs)

Disclosure: Dr M.E. Rupp reports receiving research funding and serves as a consultant for 3M and serves as a consultant for Citius Pharmaceuticals.
Division of Infectious Diseases, University of Nebraska Medical Center, 985400 Nebraska Medical Center, Omaha, NE 68198, USA
* Corresponding author.
E-mail address: merupp@unmc.edu

Infect Dis Clin N Am 32 (2018) 765–787
https://doi.org/10.1016/j.idc.2018.06.002
id.theclinics.com

from 2008 to 2014 in acute-care hospitals in the United States, tens of thousands of patients continue to experience bloodstream infection (BSI) each year, resulting in substantial morbidity and mortality and increased cost.[1] The mean rate of CLABSIs in acute-care hospital units in the United States ranges from zero to 2.9/1000 CVC days depending on the type of unit and is approximately 1/1000 CVC days in critical care units and 0.7/1000 CVC days on other inpatient units.[2]

The rate of CLABSIs in Western European hospitals is generally comparable to that based on data reported by the US National Healthcare Safety Network (NHSN). Among patients in European ICUs, 3.7% develop BSIs (1.9/1000 patient days), with 43.6% of these BSIs attributed to IV catheters.[3] Unfortunately, the incidence of CLAB-SIs in limited-resource countries is substantially higher (1.6–44.6/1000 CVC days).[4]

An estimated 30,000 to 40,000 episodes of CLABSI continue to occur in US acute-care hospitals yearly, and thousands of additional cases undoubtedly occur in other health care settings (eg, dialysis units, critical access hospitals, long-term acute-care hospitals, and long-term care facilities) that are less well defined.[1,5] CLABSI is associated with significantly increased odds of death (odds ratio 2.75; 95% CI, 1.86–4.07) and an estimated attributable cost of $45,814 (95% CI, $30,919–$65,245).[5,6]

DEFINITIONS AND SURVEILLANCE

Two major designations are used to define BSIs due to vascular catheters: CLABSIs and catheter-related bloodstream infections (CRBSIs). Although the 2 terms are often used interchangeably, they have distinct differences. CLABSI is a surveillance definition that identifies patients with a CVC who experience a BSI that is not attributable to another source.[7] CRBSI is a clinical definition that generally requires specialized microbiologic data (eg, catheter tip culture, quantitative blood cultures, and differential time to positivity [DTP] determination). The CLABSI definition by design is highly sensitive but not as highly specific. The Centers for Medicaid and Medicaid Services requires reporting of CLABSIs and has instituted financial penalties for institutions with CLABSI rates above an arbitrary threshold. Despite improvements, the CLABSI definition over-estimates the true incidence of infection and remains somewhat subjective in assigning the source of infection.[8] Furthermore, many institutions acknowledge use of an adjudication system in defining CLABSI.[9] A more robust means to validate CLABSI data is needed, and consideration should be given to monitoring all-cause BSIs to better avoid systematic under-reporting of CLABSIs or cost shifting to secondary bacteremia designations. In addition, bacteremia due to other vascular catheters (midline catheters [MCs], arterial lines, and peripheral IV catheters) should be captured in any comprehensive surveillance system designed to monitor and diminish BSIs due to IV catheters. Finally, surveillance should be extended to various non–acute-care settings.

IV catheter infections are further defined by the site and extent of infection and can involve the exit site (erythema and/or induration extending no more than 2 cm from the exit site), the tunnel track (evidence of inflammation along the subcutaneous tunnel of an implanted CVC) (**Fig. 1**), or the subcutaneous reservoir of an implanted port (**Fig. 2**). Although purulence at the insertion site (**Fig. 3**) is pathognomonic of an infected IV catheter, most CVCs that are responsible for BSIs are innocuous in appearance, and physical examination findings lack sensitivity.[10,11]

PATHOGENESIS

Fig. 4 illustrates the main routes microbes take to infect a vascular catheter. For short-term, nontunneled catheters, the dermal surface often serves as the source of

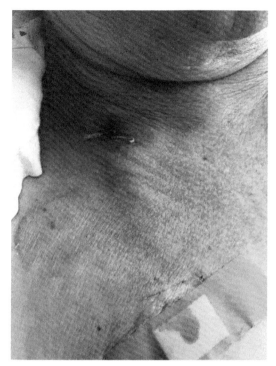

Fig. 1. Subcutaneously tunneled CVC tunnel track infection resulting in CRBSI.

microbial contamination. For subcutaneously tunneled catheters and the longer a temporary catheter stays in place, the hub and luminal surface are frequently implicated as the route of inoculation. Also, as efforts to prevent external surface contamination (CVC insertion bundles and chlorhexidine dressings) are increasingly used, hub colonization seems to have become a more prominent route of infection. Catheters are rarely seeded via a hematogenous route or via installation of contaminated infusates. Once microbes gain access to the catheter surface, they quickly adhere, proliferate, aggregate, and elaborate biofilms. The biofilms contain microbes exhibiting a variety of growth and metabolic characteristics, including very quiescent persister cells and small colony variants. Infected vascular catheters exhibiting a mature biofilm-associated infection can be difficult to treat successfully with the catheter in situ,

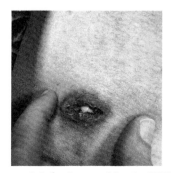

Fig. 2. Subcutaneous port reservoir infection resulting in CRBSI.

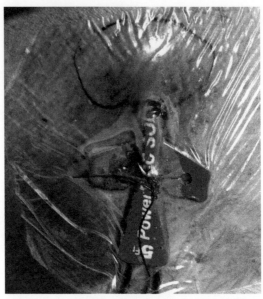

Fig. 3. Obvious purulence at the insertion site of an IV catheter in a patient with CRBSI.

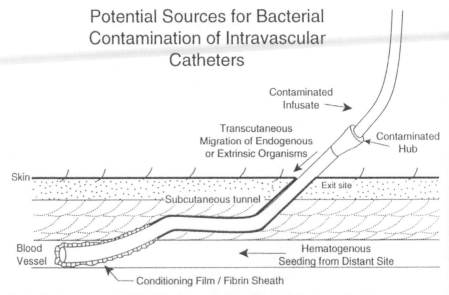

Fig. 4. Pathogenesis of CRBSI. Microbes gain access to the catheter by the following routes: external/dermal surface from transcutaneous migration and internal/luminal surface from contamination of the catheter hub, contamination of the infusate, and hematogenous seeding. (*From* Rupp ME. Infections of intravascular catheters. In: Crossley KB, Archer GL, editors. The staphylococci in human disease. New York: Churchill Livingstone; 1997. p. 381; with permission.)

and most infected catheters are removed to better ensure successful treatment and clinical outcome. Improved means to preserve vascular catheters and treat through infections are needed.

DIAGNOSIS OF CATHETER-RELATED BLOODSTREAM INFECTION

It is important to make an accurate diagnosis of CRBSI because there are grave consequences associated with inaccurate or missed diagnosis, such as unnecessary catheter removal, serious procedural complications, and increased mortality and economic costs. Definitive diagnosis of CRBSI requires clinical signs of sepsis with microbiological evidence. The Infectious Diseases Society of America (IDSA) clinical practice guideline suggests 1 of the following criteria for the definitive diagnosis of CRBSI:[10]

- Growth of the same microorganism from the culture of a catheter segment by semiquantitative roll-plate method (>15 colony-forming units [CFUs]/plate) or quantitative culture by sonication method (10^2 CFUs) and percutaneously obtained peripheral blood culture
- Paired blood cultures obtained simultaneously from a catheter lumen and peripheral blood meets the criteria for CRBSI by quantitative blood cultures ($\geq$3-fold difference in CFU in blood from catheter lumen versus peripheral blood) or DTP ($\geq$2-h difference in time to positivity, catheter lumen vs peripheral)

In situations where peripheral blood cultures or culture of catheter segment cannot be performed, a possible diagnosis of CRBSI is suggested by quantitative blood cultures obtained from 2 different lumens of the catheter in which at least a 3-fold colony count difference is noted.

Catheter Segment Culture for the Diagnosis of Catheter-Related Bloodstream Infection

Maki and colleagues[12] described the utility of the roll-plate semiquantitative culture method in the diagnosis of CRBSI and this remains a frequently used microbiologic test to assess for significant catheter colonization. When a vascular catheter (venous or arterial) is removed for suspicion of CRBSI, the distal 5 cm of the catheter (catheter segment or tip) is sent for roll-plate analysis. If a pulmonary artery catheter is implicated, the introducer tip should be cultured rather than the catheter itself.[10,13] Qualitative culture of the port reservoir is recommended for the diagnosis of a subcutaneous port infection.[14] Because the luminal surface is often involved in infections of long-term catheters, the roll-plate technique (which only samples the external surface of the catheter) is associated with significant false-negative results. Quantitative culture performed after sonication or vortex washing the catheter tip is the preferred method for sampling long-term IV catheters.[15] Unfortunately, these culture techniques require removal of the catheter. Other methods to microbiologically assess the catheter with the device in situ include paired hub and exit site cultures and use of intraluminal brushes.[16–19] A particularly innovative approach to the diagnosis of catheter colonization is the use of biosensors attached to the CVC; however, economic cost of this technology is a limiting factor.[20]

Blood Culture Methods for the Diagnosis of Catheter-Related Bloodstream Infection

Paired quantitative blood cultures
A diagnosis of CRBSI can be made in appropriate clinical settings if the microorganism colony count is at least 3-fold higher in blood cultures obtained from

the CVC versus percutaneously obtained peripheral blood.[10] A meta-analysis by Safdar and colleagues[17] calculated pooled sensitivity and specificity of 8 diagnostic methods to diagnose CRBSI and found paired quantitative blood culture the most accurate, with a sensitivity of 74% to 84% and specificity of 98% to 100%.

Differential time to positivity

The DTP test depends on the use of continuously monitored blood culture systems and is based on the finding that a blood culture with a higher inoculum shows evidence of microbial growth sooner than a blood culture with a lower inoculum. If a vascular catheter is the source of bacteremia, blood sampled through the catheter should have a higher inoculum than peripheral blood and hence should yield evidence of microbial growth more quickly. A cutoff time of 2 hours is generally used for DTP evaluation, and a meta-analysis to assess the utility of DTP for the diagnosis of CRBSI documented a sensitivity of 86% to 92% and a specificity of 79% to 87%.[17,21] Accurate DTP testing requires that an equivalent amount of blood is sampled from both catheter and peripheral sources. A recent study documented, however, that blood cultures drawn from CVCs contain a significantly greater amount of blood than peripheral blood cultures; thus, this requirement for equivalent blood volumes for DTP cultures may not be met in routine practice.[22] The role of DTP for the diagnosis of catheter-related candidemia remains controversial. A retrospective study analyzing the usefulness of DTP for diagnosis of catheter-related candidemia found a DTP greater than 2 hours was 85% sensitive and 82% specific.[23] Other investigators, however, noted poor specificity (40%) associated with DTP testing for CVC-associated candidemia.[16,23]

Multilumen catheters

Current guidelines do not recommend culturing more than 1 lumen of a CVC.[10] A retrospective study noted, however, that up to 37.5% of CRBSIs can be missed if only 1 lumen of a multilumen CVC is cultured.[24] Similarly, a retrospective study by Plane and colleagues[25] found that approximately one-third of CRBSIs are missed if all lumens of the catheter are not cultured. One solution to the added cost associated of sampling all lumens separately is to pool blood drawn from all lumens into a single blood culture bottle.[26] This pooled culture technique does not define which specific lumen is infected and this information may be important if an antimicrobial lock is used in treatment (discussed later).

Molecular-Based Testing and Biomarkers for the Diagnosis of Catheter-Related Bloodstream Infection

Significant time is often required to diagnose CRBSI due to reliance on microbial growth from blood and/or catheter segments. Molecular-based rapid diagnostic testing has evolved recently for the early identification of microorganisms in BSIs, including infections stemming from vascular catheters.[27] The utilization of rapid, non–culture-based diagnostic methods has the potential to supplement conventional microbiologic diagnosis. Non–culture-based systems also may contribute new knowledge regarding microbes, potentially causing CRBSIs that are not recoverable using traditional culture-dependent methods. Biomarkers like interleukin 6, procalcitonin, C-reactive protein, and triggering receptor expressed on myeloid cells 1 (TREM-1) have also been studied for the diagnosis of BSIs. Molecular diagnostic strategies, potentially used together with biomarker identification, may lead to faster and more sensitive means to diagnosis of CRBSI.

MANAGEMENT OF CATHETER-RELATED BLOODSTREAM INFECTION

Once CRBSI is suspected, empiric antimicrobial therapy should be administered after appropriate cultures are obtained. The choice of empiric antimicrobial agent depends on the following: most likely causative pathogen, type of catheter, host characteristics, local antimicrobial susceptibility patterns, clinical stability of the patient, and presence of complications. Some considerations for appropriate antibiotic therapy are as follows:

- Empiric antibiotics should cover gram-positive organisms; intravascular vancomycin or daptomycin is recommended in health care settings due to the high prevalence of methicillin-resistant *Staphylococcus aureus* and coagulase-negative staphylococci.
- Indications for empiric antibiotics for gram-negative bacilli include the following: neutropenia, critical illness, femoral catheter–related BSI, or known gram-negative bacilli focus of infection at the time of suspected CRBSI. The choice of empiric antibiotics for gram-negative bacilli should be based on the local antimicrobial susceptibility pattern. In general, a fourth-generation cephalosporin, β-lactam/β-lactamase inhibitor combination, or carbapenem, with or without an aminoglycoside, is recommended. In critically ill patients or patients with documented recent colonization with multidrug-resistant (MDR) gram-negative bacilli, combination therapy with 2 different classes of antimicrobials against MDR gram-negative bacilli is indicated. When treating patients with gram-negative bacilli CRBSI, significant consideration should be given for the bacilli to potentially produce AmpC β-lactamase, extended-spectrum β-lactamase (ESBL), metallo-β-lactamase, or a carbapenemase.
- Indications for empiric antifungal therapy for candidemia include critically ill patients, prolonged exposure to broad-spectrum antibiotics, recent gastrointestinal surgery, femoral catheter–related BSI, hematologic malignancies, hematopoietic stem cell transplantation, solid organ transplantion, patients on total parenteral nutrition, and presence of candida colonization at multiple body sites. Echinocandins are preferred antifungal agents for empiric therapy for candidemia, particularly if local prevalence of *Candida krusei* or *Candida glabrata* infection is high or if a patient has received an azole antifungal within the preceding 3 months. **Box 1** offers a summary of treatment considerations for CRBSIs caused by specific pathogens.

Central Venous Catheter Removal

Indications for the removal of an IV catheter in the setting of a CRBSI include the following:

- Severe sepsis, infective endocarditis, septic thrombophlebitis, or persistent bacteremia for greater than 72 hours despite appropriate antimicrobial therapy
- CRBSI due to *S aureus*, MDR gram-negative bacilli, fungi, or mycobacteria
- CRBSIs due to *Micrococcus* spp or *Propionibacterium* once blood culture contamination is ruled out by repeated recovery of the pathogen from blood cultures

A randomized controlled trial in hemodynamically stable ICU patients suspected of having CRBSI compared watchful waiting (catheter removal only after confirmed bacteremia or if new hemodynamic instability) to standard of care (immediate catheter change) and showed a substantial reduction in unnecessary catheter removal without an increase in mortality associated with the watchful waiting strategy.[28] In patients

---

Box 1
Selected pathogen-specific recommendations for treatment of catheter-related bloodstream infection

Coagulase-negative staphylococci:
- Uncomplicated infection: remove catheter and treat for 5 days to 7 days. If catheter salvage is desired, treat in combination with antibiotic lock therapy for 10 days to 14 days.
- If no IV or orthotic hardware is present, repeat blood cultures after catheter removal are negative, and there is no evidence of complicated infection, observation without antibiotic administration is reasonable alternative.
- *S lugdunensis*: treat as *S aureus*.

S aureus:
- Remove catheter and treat for 2 weeks to 6 weeks.
- TEE indicted if persistent fever or bacteremia greater than 72 hours after removal of catheter. Optimal timing for TEE is 5 days to 7 days after diagnosis of bacteremia to reduce false-negative results.
- Two weeks of parenteral antibiotics is reasonable in uncomplicated CRBSI in appropriate clinical settings.
- A replacement CVC can be inserted if repeat cultures are sterile 48 hours to 72 hours after removal of the infected CVC.

Enterococcus spp:
- Short-term catheter: remove catheter and treat for 7 days to 14 days.
- Long-term catheter: catheter removal is preferred. If catheter salvage is desired, treat for 10 days to 14 days in combination with ALT.
- TEE is indicated if there are clinical or radiographic signs of infective endocarditis or there is persistent fever or bacteremia greater than 72 hours after initiation of appropriate antibiotic therapy or the patient has a prosthetic heart valve.

Other gram-positive bacteria:
- Suspected CRBSIs due to *Micrococcus* spp, *Corynebacterium* spp, *Bacillus* spp, or *Propionibacterium* spp require confirmation of true bacteremia with multiple percutaneous blood cultures.
- Catheter removal is often required as infections are difficult to eradicate

Gram-negative bacilli:
- Empiric gram-negative coverage indication: patient is neutropenic, critically ill, or there is a known focus of gram-negative infection at the time of suspected CRBSI.
- Two empiric gram-negative antibiotics are indicated if a patient is critically ill or previously defined as colonized with an MDR gram-negative bacilli.
- *Pseudomonas* or MDR gram-negative bacilli: remove catheter and treat for 10 days to 14 days.
- Other gram-negative bacilli: remove catheter and treat for 7 days to 14 days. If catheter salvage is attempted, use parenteral antibiotics in combination with ALT for 10 days to 14 days.
- Persistent fever or bacteremia greater than 72 hours despite being on appropriate antimicrobial therapy: remove catheter and look for metastatic infection and infective endocarditis.

Candida spp:
- Remove catheter. Catheter retention is associated with worse outcome.
- Candidemia with a CVC: if no other source, remove CVC and culture tip of the catheter, or exchange catheter over a guide wire and culture tip of the catheter (if CVC is colonized, removed CVC and treat for 14 days).
- Echinocandins: if high prevalence of *Candida krusei* or *Candida glabarata* or recent azole exposure.

Abbreviation: TEE, transesophageal echocardiogram.

with limited venous access, such as hemodialysis catheter (HD) patients with extensive venous thrombosis, catheter exchange over a guide wire should be considered.[29] A systemic review to compare catheter exchange over a guide wire versus new site replacement showed a trend toward increased infections but fewer mechanical complications when the catheter was exchanged over a guide wire.[30] CRBSIs due to low-virulence organisms, particularly in the setting of a high-risk for mechanical complications for new catheter insertion, can be treated with catheter exchange over a guide wire. Many experts recommend use of an antimicrobial impregnated catheter to prevent future colonization and BSIs if the catheter is exchanged over a guide wire.[10] Increasing clinic experience, however, is being accrued regarding preservation of the CVC and treatment with the CVC in situ.[31–33] This CVC preservation strategy involves use of antimicrobial locks, discussed later.

Duration of Antibiotic Therapy

Appropriate duration of antimicrobial therapy in CRBSI is based on the causative pathogen, presence of complications, and host factors. In uncomplicated CRBSI (absence of metastatic infection, endocarditis, suppurative thrombophlebitis, IV hardware, immunosuppression, and resolution of clinical and microbiological signs of infection within 72 hours of initiation of antimicrobial agent) a shorter course of antibiotics should be considered. All complicated CRBSIs require catheter removal. **Box 2** delineates the most common complications associated with CRBSIs.

Antimicrobial Lock Therapy

Often, removal of foreign material is the most desirable approach in the treatment of a foreign body–related infection. Removal of an infected CVC, however, may not be

---

Box 2
Complications of infections of intravascular catheters

Suppurative thrombophlebitis:
- Suspect suppurative thrombophlebitis if bacteremia persists greater than 72 hours despite being on appropriate antibiotic therapy. Subcutaneous thrombosed vein may present as a cordlike structure.
- Diagnosis made by imaging (ultrasound, CT, or MRI)
- May require surgical intervention and/or anticoagulation
- Remove the catheter and treat for 4 weeks to 6 weeks with parenteral antibiotics.

Persistent bacteremia:
- Persistent bacteremia without an identifiable complication indicates the need for longer courses of antibiotics (consider 4–6 weeks). In the case of *S aureus* bacteremia, if initial TEE is negative, consider repeat TEE in 5 days to 7 days.

Infective endocarditis:
- Longer course of antibiotics (4–6 weeks) and further work-up related to complications of infective endocarditis is required. May need surgical treatment.

Osteomyelitis:
- Longer course of antibiotics (6–8 weeks) is required and surgical débridement may be needed.

Local complication:
- Catheter tunnel infection and port pocket infection require catheter removal; 7 days to 10 days of parenteral antibiotics with drainage of abscess.

Abbreviation: TEE, transesophageal echocardiogram.

possible or practical for a variety of reasons, such as extremely limited alternative vascular access or unacceptable complications associated with removal and replacement. ALT is an alternative when catheter removal is not possible, or catheter salvage is desired. Although there is no Food and Drug Administration (FDA)-approved antimicrobial lock solution, ALT is recommended by many experts in adjunct to parenteral antibiotic therapy for catheter salvage.[10] The ALT solution consists of a highly concentrated antibiotic (100–1000 times the minimum inhibitory concentration), which is generally mixed with an anticoagulant.[34] Sufficient volume of the antimicrobial lock solution (usually 2 mL–5 mL) is infused to fill the catheter lumen and it is allowed to dwell in place for hours (the optimum duration of dwell time is unknown, but many institutional ALT protocols suggest a minimum of 2–4 hours). The hallmark of a vascular catheter–associated infection is the presence of a biofilm and, unfortunately, the ability of many antimicrobial agents to kill microorganisms is significantly reduced in a biofilm due to the following: decreased antimicrobial biofilm penetration, presence of inactivating enzymes and efflux pumps in biofilms, and the presence of metabolically quiescent persister cells.[35,36] Citrate and EDTA improve the activity of antimicrobial lock solutions by disrupting biofilm and improving antimicrobial biofilm penetration.[37,38] There are no commercially available ALT solutions. Properties of an ideal ALT solution include the following: intrinsic antimicrobial activity against the offending microorganism, ability to penetrate and disrupt biofilm cells, compatibility with an anticoagulant, prolonged stability, minimal risk for toxicity, low potential for resistance, compatibility with catheter materials, and cost-effectiveness.[34] A randomized double-blind placebo-controlled trial to evaluate the effect of ALT in the treatment of CRBSI in patients with long-term IV devices showed ALT reduced the failure rate from 57% to 33%.[31] Raad and colleagues[39] observed successful salvage of infected CVCs in cancer patients with use of ALT consisting of minocycline, EDTA, and 25% alcohol. A recent systemic review analyzing ALT in CRBSIs suggested that the introduction of components, such as daptomycin, tigecycline, ethanol, and taurolidine, into ALT solutions increased their effectiveness in catheter salvage.[40] **Box 3** summarizes some of the considerations regarding ALT.

PREVENTION

Methods to prevent vascular catheter infections can be broadly grouped into 2 categories: clinical practice–based measures (**Box 4**) and technologic approaches (**Box 5**). Several comprehensive, evidence-based guidelines have been promulgated to steer

---

Box 3
Summary of considerations regarding antimicrobial lock therapy

- Recommended as adjunct to parenteral antibiotic therapy for catheter salvage
- Antibiotic solution (100–1000 times the MIC) mixed with an anticoagulant installed in the catheter lumen and allowed to dwell for hours
- Higher rate of treatment failure with *S aureus*, *Pseudomonas*, and *Candida* infection
- Concentration of antibiotic can substantially decline over time; antibiotic lock solution should be changed at least every 48 hours.
- Infections occurring shortly after catheter insertion (less than 2 weeks) are often extraluminal; ALT is not likely beneficial.

Abbreviation: MIC, minimum inhibitory concentration.

Box 4
Evidence-based practice interventions (human behavior–oriented interventions) to prevent catheter-related bloodstream infections

Pericatheter insertion
  Appropriate staffing
  Education and training; infusion team
  Use of maximal sterile barriers
  Insertion site selection
  Cutaneous antisepsis with chlorhexidine
  Use of insertion checklist
  Bundle approach

Postcatheter insertion
  Scrub the hub—disinfection of hubs and needleless connectors
  Chlorhexidine patient bathing
  Removal of unneeded catheters
  Catheter dressing maintenance
  Bundle approach

---

preventive techniques and the main points are summarized in the following discussion.[41–43]

Practice-Based Interventions

Staffing and education

Experience from several CRBSI outbreaks indicates that when units are not staffed with stable and well-trained personnel (nurses and physicians), optimum infection prevention procedures and protocols are not maintained and excess health care–associated infections are the result.[44–46] It is difficult to stipulate minimum staffing requirements from an infection prevention viewpoint because patient acuity and staffing needs vary from unit to unit and from day to day. It suffices to state that units should be staffed with an adequate number of personnel and the personnel must be appropriately educated and trained with regard to vascular catheter selection, proper insertion procedures, catheter care and maintenance, and catheter removal. Some institutions have successfully decreased CLABSI rates by instituting specially trained teams to insert and care for CVCs.[43] There is also a growing recognition that the patient and patient's family should be included in IV catheter education, particularly if they are involved in out-of-hospital care.[42,47]

Box 5
Evidence-based technologic innovation interventions (new devices and technology) to prevent catheter-related bloodstream infections

Antimicrobial catheter coatings (silver-sulfadiazine/chlorhexidine or minocycline/rifampin)

Chlorhexidine-impregnated dressings (sponge dressing or gel pad dressing)

Passive port protectors

Silver-impregnated connectors

Sutureless catheter securement

Antimicrobial catheter locks

Maximal sterile barrier precautions and checklist

Maximal sterile barrier precautions should be used for the insertion of all CVCs and consist of sterile gloves, long-sleeved sterile gown, cap, procedure mask, and a long sterile drape that covers the patient from head to toe.[48,49] To ensure compliance with appropriate insertion procedures, a bedside checklist should be used.[50] A person other than the CVC inserter should complete the checklist and the observer should be empowered to stop the procedure if violations in aseptic technique are noted.

Chlorhexidine cutaneous antiseptic

In patients without contraindications (eg, chlorhexidine allergy), the skin should be disinfected with an alcoholic chlorhexidine solution containing at least 0.5% chlorhexidine.[51] The insertion site should be allowed to dry before catheter insertion. Increasing data indicate that chlorhexidine can be used safely for skin disinfection in some groups of neonates.[52,53]

Insertion site

The femoral site may be more prone to colonization and infection, particularly in obese patients, and should thus be avoided.[54] Although the subclavian site seems the least prone to infectious complications, due to ease of placement with the use of ultrasound guidance, the internal jugular site is often preferred by clinicians.[55–57] In all cases, the CVC insertion site should be individualized and depends on experience of the operator, risk of complications, anticipated duration of catheterization, potential need for dialysis, and other patient factors.[57]

Bundle

A variety of prevention measures can be combined to create a bundle. In many institutions, the bundle consists of use of an all-inclusive insertion kit or catheter cart, hand hygiene, use of alcoholic chlorhexidine for skin disinfection, avoidance of the femoral site, use of maximal sterile barrier precautions, and removal of CVCs as soon as practical.[58,59] The relative contribution of elements of the bundle has not been defined and this approach is most successful when used in a multidisciplinary manner in an institution with a good patient safety foundation.

Postinsertion precautions

As increasing numbers of institutions have instituted peri-insertion checklists and bundles, contamination of the CVC at the time of insertion has become less frequent and a shift in CLABSI etiology away from commensal skin organisms has been evident.[60] This points to the increasing importance of post-CVC insertion preventive measures.

Removal of unneeded or potentially contaminated central venous catheters

The need for CVCs should be assessed daily and unnecessary CVCs should be removed. Programmatic approaches to CVC assessment and removal are most effective if they use a standardized procedure and use checklists, audits, and electronic monitoring and reminders.[54,61] Also, in instances in which compliance with CVC insertion precautions cannot be assured (emergent CVC insertion in the field or code blue situations), the CVC should be removed and replaced at a new site as soon as a patient's condition allows (within 24–48 hours).[41,43]

Catheter hub and needleless connector disinfection—"scrub the hub"

An appropriate antiseptic (70% alcohol, alcoholic chlorhexidine, and povidone iodine) should be used to scrub the catheter hub or needleless connector before accessing the catheter. The minimum scrub time to adequately disinfect needleless connectors is not defined and depends on the connector design and degree of contamination.[62] It seems that some connector designs are associated with a greater risk of BSI and this probably relates to features, such as transparency, displacement, fluid pathway and flow dynamics, and, perhaps most important, the ease of cleaning of the interface between the diaphragm and the plastic housing (smooth, easy-to clean interface without cracks or crevices).[63–65]

Chlorhexidine patient bathing
Chlorhexidine is believed a more effective disinfectant to prevent CLABSI due to its long residual activity and resistance to inactivation.[66] As discussed previously, chlorhexidine should be used for skin disinfection for initial CVC insertion and then routinely during dressing changes.[41–43] In addition, a growing body of literature indicates that routine patient bathing with chlorhexidine or universal decolonization protocols results in CLABSI prevention.[67–70] There is concern, however, that widespread or indiscriminate use of chlorhexidine will promote the emergence of chlorhexidine resistance.[71]

Catheter dressing integrity and administration set replacement
CVC dressings should be changed at weekly intervals for transparent semipermeable dressings and every 2 days for gauze dressings.[41–43] Dressing integrity seems to be an important risk factor for the development of CLABSIs, and CVC dressings should be changed whenever they become loose, damp, or soiled.[41–43,72] Because frequent administration set change does not decrease CLABSIs, administration sets should be routinely changed no more frequently than every 96 hours.[43] Administration sets for parenteral nutrition should be changed every 24 hours, whereas those used to administer blood and blood products should be changed after the completion of each unit or every 4 hours.[43] Tubing for propofol infusions should be changed every 6 hours to 12 hours.[43] Disconnection/reconnection of infusion sets should be minimized.

Postinsertion bundles
Many institutions have combined postinsertion measures to prevent CLABSIs into bundles consisting of reminders to remove CVCs and compliance with scrub-the-hub and dressing integrity recommendations.[73,74]

Technologic Innovations to Prevent Catheter-Related Bloodstream Infection
In recent years, a variety of innovative devices designed to prevent CRBSIs have been brought to market (see **Box 5**). In some instances, because human behavior can be difficult to change, the introduction of a device that protects against lapses in human practices (hand hygiene, scrub the hub, appropriate CVC dressing changes, and so forth) may be particularly useful and cost effective. The following section briefly covers commercially available products.

Antimicrobial coated intravascular catheters
There is extensive experience and a large body of evidence to indicate that CVCs coated with antimicrobial agents are associated with a decreased risk of CRBSI.[75–78] The catheters with the greatest amount of supporting data are coated with either silver sulfadiazine/chlorhexidine or minocycline/rifampin. Fewer data are available to support use of CVCs with other coatings.[75,78] Available data suggest that use of antimicrobial coated CVCs does not result in an emergence of antibiotic resistance.[79] Guidelines suggest that antimicrobial coated CVCs be used in patients in whom the catheter is expected to stay in place at least 5 days and when routine practice measures (ie, insertion bundle and postinsertion care) have not eliminated preventable

CRBSI.[41–43] These considerations, however, are appropriate for all technologic approaches to CRBSI prevention.

Chlorhexidine-impregnated dressings
Chlorhexidine-impregnated dressings prevent microorganisms present at the skin and the insertion site from proliferating and gaining access to the external surface of the CVC. Extensive data exist supporting their use to prevent CRBSIs.[72,80]

Antibiotic-impregnated needleless connectors
Needleless connectors may be prone to microbial colonization resulting in BSIs. To decrease this risk, connectors impregnated with silver have been introduced. Silver-impregnated connectors are less prone to microbial colonization, and their use may decrease CRBSIs.[81,82]

Passive port protectors
As discussed previously, the widespread use of insertion precautions to prevent contamination and chlorhexidine skin disinfection with dressing changes or patient bathing regimens has resulted in a shift in the most prominent route of inoculation from the external/dermal surface of the CVC to the hub/luminal surface. Because it is difficult to maintain strict aseptic technique with all CVC access events, some institutions have introduced passive port protectors that bathe the catheter connector hub with alcohol when it is not in use. There are increasing data that this is an effective means to prevent CRBSIs.[83,84]

Catheter lock solutions
Although there are no FDA-approved catheter lock solutions for the prevention or treatment of CRBSIs, there is a great amount of data to indicate that antibiotic or antiseptic solutions can be used to prevent CRBSIs.[85–88] A variety of antibiotics and antiseptics have been used in solutions to lock catheters, and antimicrobial locks are increasingly used to prevent infections in patients with long-term need for vascular access (hemodialysis, total parenteral nutrition dependence, and so forth) or in patients with a history of recurrent CRBSI.

Catheter securement
Sutures used to secure CVCs result in trauma to the skin and provide a foreign body nidus for microbial colonization.[89] Therefore, sutureless securement systems have been developed and are supported by some clinical data.[90,91]

CONSIDERATIONS REGARDING OTHER VASCULAR CATHETERS
Peripheral Intravascular Catheters

Peripheral intravascular catheters (PIVCs) are nearly ubiquitous in hospitalized patients, and approximately 330 million PIVCs are purchased in the United States yearly.[92–94] The incidence of PIVC-BSI is approximately 0.2% and approximately 20% of S aureus BSIs are due to infected PIVCs.[94] At present, because of their widespread use and limited appreciation of risk, as well as successful programs to prevent CRBSIs, there may be more patients experiencing BSIs due to PIVCs than due to CVCs.[94] Prolonged PIVC dwell time seems directly related to the risk of colonization and infection.[94] At present, many institutions recommend that PIVCs are replaced every 3 days to 4 days.[41] There is a growing body of evidence, however, that PIVCs can be changed based on clinical indications rather than on a set schedule and the PIVC dwell time will most likely increase.[95,96] Therefore, it will become increasingly important for institutions to develop standardized programs to ensure that personnel inserting PIVCs are competent and that PIVCs are inspected daily and removed with evidence of phlebitis or exudate. In addition, similar to CVCs, PVICs that are inserted emergently or without appropriate aseptic technique should be replaced as soon as practical.

Midline Catheters

MCs, generally composed of polyurethane or silicone and 8 cm to 20 cm in length, are usually placed proximal to the antecubital fossa with the tip terminating below the axillary vein. MCs are FDA approved for short-term vascular access of less than 30 days. Adverse reactions and hypersensitivity due to catheter materials resulted in a decline in use of MCs in the 1990s.[97,98] In more recent years, however, with changes in catheter materials and design, a resurgence in use of MCs is evident. Besides their longer duration of use compared with PIVCs, MCs have the advantage of being compatible with power injection and can be multilumen. Because they are located in the peripheral vein, they do not require radiographic confirmation regarding placement location. MCs are not compatible with infusates of high osmolality or pH outside the 5 to 9 range.[99] Increasing experience indicates, however, that medications outside these parameters can be safely administered via MCs.[99,100]

There are few data regarding complications of MCs. It seems they are less likely to result in BSIs than CVCs, and available studies report BSI rates less than 0.5/1000 MC days.[99,101,102] Other complications, however, such as phlebitis and thrombosis, seem more common in MCs than CVCs.[92,99,101] Because BSIs due to PIVCs and MCs do not count as a CLABSIs and because mechanical complications are generally not tracked or reported to regulatory agencies, some institutions are relying heavily on MCs to limit the use of CVCs and thus decrease CLABSIs.

Arterial Catheters

Most studies conclude that ACs are associated with about the same risk of BSIs as nontunneled CVCs.[103–109] ACs, however, are often regarded as less infection prone and they are generally not included in surveillance programs that track CLABSIs. Femoral ACs may be more prone to BSIs than other sites and the femoral site should be avoided if possible.[106,109] ACs should be inserted and cared for with the same level of concern as CVCs. Unfortunately, surveys suggest that aseptic technique and appropriate barrier precautions are often violated when ACs are inserted.[110]

Hemodialysis Catheters

Compared with patients receiving HD via an arteriovenous fistula or graft, those undergoing HD via an IV catheter are more likely to experience CRBSI. Tunneled HD catheters are less prone to infection than nontunneled HD catheters. In the 2014 Centers for Disease Control and Prevention NHSN Dialysis Event Surveillance Report,[111] 6005 outpatient dialysis facilities in the United States reported a total of 22,576 dialysis access–related BSIs, of which 69.8% were associated with CVCs. HD catheter–associated BSIs can be prevented by application of antimicrobial ointment at the catheter exit site as well as weekly administration of recombinant tissue plasminogen activating factor.[112–114] In diagnosis of HD catheter–associated BSIs, poor peripheral access may preclude collection of peripheral blood cultures and thus blood cultures from HD bloodline are often relied on. Specific recommendations regarding the treatment of HD catheter–associated BSIs follow:

- HD catheter removal is indicated when infection is due to *S aureus, Pseudomonas* spp, or *Candida* spp.

- BSIs due to gram-negative bacilli (other than *Pseudomonas* spp) and coagulase-negative staphylococci can be empirically treated with systemic antibiotics without immediate removal of HD catheter. If significant clinical improvement within 48 hours to 72 hours is not observed, catheter exchange over a guide wire is appropriate.
- HD catheters should be removed in the presence of metastatic infections, persistent fever, or bacteremia for greater than 72 hours despite appropriate antimicrobial treatment.
- Treatment with parenteral antibiotics in combination with ALT can be done if there is clinical improvement within 48 hours to 72 hours and there is no absolute indication to remove the HD catheter, as discussed previously.

SUMMARY

Despite the great strides that have been made in recent years to prevent CRBSI, it remains a significant clinical problem. Emphasis should continue to be placed on practice-based measures, such as education, training, and application of insertion and maintenance bundles. Elimination of preventable CRBSIs, however, also requires judicious use of technologic innovations, such as coated catheters and impregnated dressings. It is evident that many catheter infections can be successfully treated with the catheter in situ through the application of antimicrobial locks—however, patient selection remains undefined and an approved catheter lock solution is lacking. Important questions remain regarding all facets of CRBSI—including pathogenesis, diagnosis and surveillance, prevention, and treatment.

ACKNOWLEDGMENTS

The authors thank Sandy Nelson for expert assistance in preparation of this article.

REFERENCES

1. Centers for Disease Control and Prevention (CDC). National and state healthcare associated infections progress report. Available at: http://www.cdc.gov/HAI/pdfs/progress-report/hai-progress-report.pdf. Accessed July 26, 2018.
2. Dudeck MA, Edwards JR, Allen-Bridson K, et al. National healthcare safety network report, data summary for 2013, device-associated module. Am J Infect Control 2015;43(3):206–21.
3. European Centre for Disease Prevention and Control. Healthcare-associated infections acquired in intensive care units. In: ECDC, editor. Annual epidemiological report for 2016. Stockholm: ECDC; 2018.
4. Rosenthal VD. Central line-associated bloodstream infections in limited-resource countries: a review of the literature. Clin Infect Dis 2009;49(12):1899–907.
5. Zimlichman E, Henderson D, Tamir O, et al. Health care-associated infections: a meta-analysis of costs and financial impact on the US health care system. JAMA Intern Med 2013;173(22):2039–46.
6. Ziegler MJ, Pellegrini DC, Safdar N. Attributable mortality of central line associated bloodstream infection: systematic review and meta-analysis. Infection 2015;43(1):29–36.
7. Centers for Disease Control and Prevention. National healthcare safety network (NHSN) patient safety component manual. Chapter 4: Bloodstream infection

event (central line-associated bloodstream infection and non-central line associated bloodstream infection). 2018. Available at: https://www.cdc.gov/nhsn/pdfs/pscmanual/pcsmanualcurrent.pdf. Accessed July 26, 2018.

8. Mayer J, Greene T, Howell J, et al. Agreement in classifying bloodstream infections among multiple reviewers conducting surveillance. Clin Infect Dis 2012; 55(3):364–70.

9. Beekmann SE, Diekema DJ, Huskins WC, et al. Diagnosing and reporting of central line-associated bloodstream infections. Infect Control Hosp Epidemiol 2012;33(9):875–82.

10. Mermel LA, Allon M, Bouza E, et al. Clinical practice guidelines for the diagnosis and management of intravascular catheter-related infection: 2009 update by the infectious diseases society of america. Clin Infect Dis 2009;49(1):1–45.

11. Safdar N, Maki DG. Inflammation at the insertion site is not predictive of catheter-related bloodstream infection with short-term, noncuffed central venous catheters. Crit Care Med 2002;30(12):2632–5.

12. Maki D, Weise C, Sarafin H. A semiquantitative culture method for identifying intravenous-catheter-related infection. N Engl J Med 1977;296:1305–9.

13. Mermel LA, McCormick RD, Springman SR, et al. The pathogenesis and epidemiology of catheter-related infection with pulmonary artery swan-ganz catheters: a prospective study utilizing molecular subtyping. Am J Med 1991; 91(3B):197S–205S.

14. Douard MC, Arlet G, Longuet P, et al. Diagnosis of venous access port-related infections. Clin Infect Dis 1999;29(5):1197–202.

15. Slobbe L, El Barzouhi A, Boersma E, et al. Comparison of the roll plate method to the sonication method to diagnose catheter colonization and bacteremia in patients with long-term tunnelled catheters: a randomized prospective study. J Clin Microbiol 2009;47(4):885–8.

16. Bouza E, Alvarado N, Alcala L, et al. A prospective, randomized, and comparative study of 3 different methods for the diagnosis of intravascular catheter colonization. Clin Infect Dis 2005;40(8):1096–100.

17. Safdar N, Fine JP, Maki DG. Meta-analysis: methods for diagnosing intravascular device-related bloodstream infection. Ann Intern Med 2005;142(6): 451–66.

18. Cercenado E, Ena J, Rodriguez-Creixems M, et al. A conservative procedure for the diagnosis of catheter-related infections. Arch Intern Med 1990;150(7): 1417–20.

19. Catton JA, Dobbins BM, Kite P, et al. In situ diagnosis of intravascular catheter-related bloodstream infection: a comparison of quantitative culture, differential time to positivity, and endoluminal brushing. Crit Care Med 2005;33(4):787–91.

20. Paredes J, Alonso-Arce M, Schmidt C, et al. Smart central venous port for early detection of bacterial biofilm related infections. Biomed Microdevices 2014; 16(3):365–74.

21. Raad I, Hanna HA, Alakech B, et al. Differential time to positivity: a useful method for diagnosing catheter-related bloodstream infections. Ann Intern Med 2004;140(1):18–25.

22. Jones RL, Sayles HR, Fey PD, et al. Effect of clinical variables on the volume of blood collected for blood cultures in an adult patient population. Infect Control Hosp Epidemiol 2017;38(12):1493–7.

23. Park KH, Lee MS, Lee SO, et al. Diagnostic usefulness of differential time to positivity for catheter-related candidemia. J Clin Microbiol 2014;52(7): 2566–72.

24. Guembe M, Rodriguez-Creixems M, Sanchez-Carrillo C, et al. How many lumens should be cultured in the conservative diagnosis of catheter-related bloodstream infections? Clin Infect Dis 2010;50(12):1575–9.

25. Planes AM, Calleja R, Bernet A, et al. Evaluation of the usefulness of a quantitative blood culture in the diagnosis of catheter-related bloodstream infection: comparative analysis of two periods (2002 and 2012). Enferm Infecc Microbiol Clin 2016;34(8):484–9.

26. Herrera-Guerra AS, Garza-Gonzalez E, Martinez-Resendez MF, et al. Individual versus pooled multiple-lumen blood cultures for the diagnosis of intravascular catheter-related infections. Am J Infect Control 2015;43(7):715–8.

27. Zhang L, Rickard CM. Non-culture based diagnostics for intravascular catheter related bloodstream infections. Expert Rev Mol Diagn 2017;17(2):181–8.

28. Rijnders BJ, Peetermans WE, Verwaest C, et al. Watchful waiting versus immediate catheter removal in ICU patients with suspected catheter-related infection: a randomized trial. Intensive Care Med 2004;30(6):1073–80.

29. Casey J, Davies J, Balshaw-Greer A, et al. Inserting tunnelled hemodialysis catheters using elective guidewire exchange from nontunnelled catheters: is there a greater risk of infection when compared with new-site replacement? Hemodial Int 2008;12(1):52–4.

30. Cook D, Randolph A, Kernerman P, et al. Central venous catheter replacement strategies: a systematic review of the literature. Crit Care Med 1997;25(8):1417–24.

31. Rijnders BJ, Van Wijngaerden E, Vandecasteele SJ, et al. Treatment of long-term intravascular catheter-related bacteraemia with antibiotic lock: randomized, placebo-controlled trial. J Antimicrob Chemother 2005;55(1):90–4.

32. Fortun J, Grill F, Martin-Davila P, et al. Treatment of long-term intravascular catheter-related bacteraemia with antibiotic-lock therapy. J Antimicrob Chemother 2006;58(4):816–21.

33. Sanchez-Munoz A, Aguado JM, Lopez-Martin A, et al. Usefulness of antibiotic-lock technique in management of oncology patients with uncomplicated bacteremia related to tunneled catheters. Eur J Clin Microbiol Infect Dis 2005;24(4):291–3.

34. Justo JA, Bookstaver PB. Antibiotic lock therapy: review of technique and logistical challenges. Infect Drug Resist 2014;7:343–63.

35. Lewis K, Spoering A, Kaldalu N, et al. Persisters: specialized cells responsible for biofilm tolerance to antimicrobial agents [Chapter: 12]. In: Pace JL, Rupp ME, Finch RG, editors. Biofilms, infection, and antimicrobial therapy. Boca Raton (FL): Taylor & Francis; 2006. p. 241–53.

36. Georgopapadakou N. Antibiotic resistance in biofilms [Chapter: 21]. In: Pace JL, Rupp ME, Finch RG, editors. Biofilms, infection, and antimicrobial therapy. Boca Raton (FL): Taylor & Francis; 2006. p. 401–5.

37. Banin E, Brady KM, Greenberg EP. Chelator-induced dispersal and killing of pseudomonas aeruginosa cells in a biofilm. Appl Environ Microbiol 2006;72(3):2064–9.

38. Raad II, Fang X, Keutgen XM, et al. The role of chelators in preventing biofilm formation and catheter-related bloodstream infections. Curr Opin Infect Dis 2008;21(4):385–92.

39. Raad I, Chaftari AM, Zakhour R, et al. Successful salvage of central venous catheters in patients with catheter-related or central line-associated bloodstream infections by using a catheter lock solution consisting of

minocycline, EDTA, and 25% ethanol. Antimicrob Agents Chemother 2016; 60(6):3426–32.

40. Vassallo M, Dunais B, Roger PM. Antimicrobial lock therapy in central-line associated bloodstream infections: a systematic review. Infection 2015;43(4): 389–98.

41. O'Grady NP, Alexander M, Burns LA, et al. Guidelines for the prevention of intravascular catheter-related infections. Am J Infect Control 2011;39(4 Suppl 1): S1–34.

42. Marschall J, Mermel LA, Fakih M, et al. Strategies to prevent central line-associated bloodstream infections in acute care hospitals: 2014 update. Infect Control Hosp Epidemiol 2014;35(Suppl 2):S89–107.

43. Gorski L, Hadaway L, Hagle M, et al. Infusion therapy. Standards of practice. J Infus Nurs 2016;39(15):S17–8.

44. Fridkin SK, Pear SM, Williamson TH, et al. The role of understaffing in central venous catheter-associated bloodstream infections. Infect Control Hosp Epidemiol 1996;17(3):150–8.

45. Stone PW, Pogorzelska M, Kunches L, et al. Hospital staffing and health care-associated infections: a systematic review of the literature. Clin Infect Dis 2008;47(7):937–44.

46. Leistner R, Thurnagel S, Schwab F, et al. The impact of staffing on central venous catheter associated bloodstream infections in preterm neonates - results of nation-wide cohort study in germany. Antimicrob Resist Infect Control 2013;2(1):11.

47. Nailon R, Rupp ME. A community collaborative to develop consensus guidelines to standardize out-of-hospital maintenance care of central venous catheters. J Infus Nurs 2015;38(2):115–21.

48. Raad II, Hohn DC, Gilbreath BJ, et al. Prevention of central venous catheter-related infections by using maximal sterile barrier precautions during insertion. Infect Control Hosp Epidemiol 1994;15(4 Pt 1):231–8.

49. Hu KK, Veenstra DL, Lipsky BA, et al. Use of maximal sterile barriers during central venous catheter insertion: clinical and economic outcomes. Clin Infect Dis 2004;39(10):1441–5.

50. Berenholtz SM, Pronovost PJ, Lipsett PA, et al. Eliminating catheter-related bloodstream infections in the intensive care unit. Crit Care Med 2004;32(10): 2014–20.

51. Chaiyakunapruk N, Veenstra DL, Lipsky BA, et al. Chlorhexidine compared with povidone-iodine solution for vascular catheter-site care: a meta-analysis. Ann Intern Med 2002;136(11):792–801.

52. Chapman AK, Aucott SW, Milstone AM. Safety of chlorhexidine gluconate used for skin antisepsis in the preterm infant. J Perinatol 2012;32(1):4–9.

53. Sathiyamurthy S, Banerjee J, Godambe SV. Antiseptic use in the neonatal intensive care unit - a dilemma in clinical practice: an evidence based review. World J Clin Pediatr 2016;5(2):159–71.

54. Parenti CM, Lederle FA, Impola CL, et al. Reduction of unnecessary intravenous catheter use. internal medicine house staff participate in a successful quality improvement project. Arch Intern Med 1994;154(16):1829–32.

55. Merrer J, De Jonghe B, Golliot F, et al. Complications of femoral and subclavian venous catheterization in critically ill patients: a randomized controlled trial. JAMA 2001;286(6):700–7.

56. Randolph AG, Cook DJ, Gonzales CA, et al. Ultrasound guidance for placement of central venous catheters: a meta-analysis of the literature. Crit Care Med 1996;24(12):2053–8.

57. Marik PE, Flemmer M, Harrison W. The risk of catheter-related bloodstream infection with femoral venous catheters as compared to subclavian and internal jugular venous catheters: a systematic review of the literature and meta-analysis. Crit Care Med 2012;40(8):2479–85.

58. Pronovost P, Needham D, Berenholtz S, et al. An intervention to decrease catheter-related bloodstream infections in the ICU. N Engl J Med 2006; 355(26):2725–32.

59. Blot K, Bergs J, Vogelaers D, et al. Prevention of central line-associated bloodstream infections through quality improvement interventions: a systematic review and meta-analysis. Clin Infect Dis 2014;59(1):96–105.

60. Zakhour R, Chaftari AM, Raad II. Catheter-related infections in patients with haematological malignancies: novel preventive and therapeutic strategies. Lancet Infect Dis 2016;16(11):e241–50.

61. Seguin P, Laviolle B, Isslame S, et al. Effectiveness of simple daily sensitization of physicians to the duration of central venous and urinary tract catheterization. Intensive Care Med 2010;36(7):1202–6.

62. Rupp ME, Yu S, Huerta T, et al. Adequate disinfection of a split-septum needleless intravascular connector with a 5-second alcohol scrub. Infect Control Hosp Epidemiol 2012;33(7):661–5.

63. Rupp ME, Sholtz LA, Jourdan DR, et al. Outbreak of bloodstream infection temporally associated with the use of an intravascular needleless valve. Clin Infect Dis 2007;44(11):1408–14.

64. Jarvis WR, Murphy C, Hall KK, et al. Health care-associated bloodstream infections associated with negative- or positive-pressure or displacement mechanical valve needleless connectors. Clin Infect Dis 2009;49(12):1821–7.

65. Tabak YP, Jarvis WR, Sun X, et al. Meta-analysis on central line-associated bloodstream infections associated with a needleless intravenous connector with a new engineering design. Am J Infect Control 2014;42(12):1278–84.

66. Denton G. Chlorhexidine. In: Block SS, editor. Disinfection, sterilization, and preservation. 5th edition. Philadelphia: Lippincott Williams & Wilkins; 2001. p. 321–33.

67. Huang SS, Septimus E, Kleinman K, et al. Targeted versus universal decolonization to prevent ICU infection. N Engl J Med 2013;368(24):2255–65.

68. Climo MW, Yokoe DS, Warren DK, et al. Effect of daily chlorhexidine bathing on hospital-acquired infection. N Engl J Med 2013;368(6):533–42.

69. Kim HY, Lee WK, Na S, et al. The effects of chlorhexidine gluconate bathing on health care-associated infection in intensive care units: a meta-analysis. J Crit Care 2016;32:126–37.

70. Frost SA, Alogso MC, Metcalfe L, et al. Chlorhexidine bathing and health care-associated infections among adult intensive care patients: a systematic review and meta-analysis. Crit Care 2016;20(1):379.

71. Kampf G. Acquired resistance to chlorhexidine - is it time to establish an 'antiseptic stewardship' initiative? J Hosp Infect 2016;94(3):213–27.

72. Timsit JF, Mimoz O, Mourvillier B, et al. Randomized controlled trial of chlorhexidine dressing and highly adhesive dressing for preventing catheter-related infections in critically ill adults. Am J Respir Crit Care Med 2012;186(12):1272–8.

73. Exline MC, Ali NA, Zikri N, et al. Beyond the bundle–journey of a tertiary care medical intensive care unit to zero central line-associated bloodstream infections. Crit Care 2013;17(2):R41.

74. Guerin K, Wagner J, Rains K, et al. Reduction in central line-associated bloodstream infections by implementation of a postinsertion care bundle. Am J Infect Control 2010;38(6):430–3.

75. Casey AL, Mermel LA, Nightingale P, et al. Antimicrobial central venous catheters in adults: a systematic review and meta-analysis. Lancet Infect Dis 2008; 8(12):763–76.

76. Lai NM, Chaiyakunapruk N, Lai NA, et al. Catheter impregnation, coating or bonding for reducing central venous catheter-related infections in adults. Cochrane Database Syst Rev 2016;(3):CD007878.

77. Ramritu P, Halton K, Collignon P, et al. A systematic review comparing the relative effectiveness of antimicrobial-coated catheters in intensive care units. Am J Infect Control 2008;36(2):104–17.

78. Wang H, Huang T, Jing J, et al. Effectiveness of different central venous catheters for catheter-related infections: a network meta-analysis. J Hosp Infect 2010; 76(1):1–11.

79. Ramos ER, Reitzel R, Jiang Y, et al. Clinical effectiveness and risk of emerging resistance associated with prolonged use of antibiotic-impregnated catheters: more than 0.5 million catheter days and 7 years of clinical experience. Crit Care Med 2011;39(2):245–51.

80. Timsit JF, Bouadma L, Ruckly S, et al. Dressing disruption is a major risk factor for catheter-related infections. Crit Care Med 2012;40(6):1707–14.

81. Casey AL, Karpanen TJ, Nightingale P, et al. Microbiological comparison of a silver-coated and a non-coated needleless intravascular connector in clinical use. J Hosp Infect 2012;80(4):299–303.

82. Jacob JT, Chernetsky Tejedor S, Dent Reyes M, et al. Comparison of a silver-coated needleless connector and a standard needleless connector for the prevention of central line-associated bloodstream infections. Infect Control Hosp Epidemiol 2015;36(3):294–301.

83. Wright MO, Tropp J, Schora DM, et al. Continuous passive disinfection of catheter hubs prevents contamination and bloodstream infection. Am J Infect Control 2013;41(1):33–8.

84. Kamboj M, Blair R, Bell N, et al. Use of disinfection cap to reduce central-line-associated bloodstream infection and blood culture contamination among hematology-oncology patients. Infect Control Hosp Epidemiol 2015;36(12): 1401–8.

85. Zacharioudakis IM, Zervou FN, Arvanitis M, et al. Antimicrobial lock solutions as a method to prevent central line-associated bloodstream infections: a meta-analysis of randomized controlled trials. Clin Infect Dis 2014;59(12):1741–9.

86. Snaterse M, Ruger W, Scholte Op Reimer WJ, et al. Antibiotic-based catheter lock solutions for prevention of catheter-related bloodstream infection: a systematic review of randomised controlled trials. J Hosp Infect 2010;75(1):1–11.

87. Oliveira C, Nasr A, Brindle M, et al. Ethanol locks to prevent catheter-related bloodstream infections in parenteral nutrition: a meta-analysis. Pediatrics 2012;129(2):318–29.

88. Maiefski M, Rupp ME, Hermsen ED. Ethanol lock technique: review of the literature. Infect Control Hosp Epidemiol 2009;30(11):1096–108.

89. Karpanen TJ, Casey AL, Whitehouse T, et al. Clinical evaluation of a chlorhexidine intravascular catheter gel dressing on short-term central venous catheters. Am J Infect Control 2016;44(1):54–60.

90. Yamamoto AJ, Solomon JA, Soulen MC, et al. Sutureless securement device reduces complications of peripherally inserted central venous catheters. J Vasc Interv Radiol 2002;13(1):77–81.

91. Ullman AJ, Cooke ML, Mitchell M, et al. Dressings and securement devices for central venous catheters (CVC). Cochrane Database Syst Rev 2015;(9):CD010367.

92. Mushtaq A, Navalkele B, Kaur M, et al. Comparison of midline vs. central venous catheter-related bloodstream infections: are midlines safer than central venous lines? Open Forum Infect Dis 2017;4(1):S637. Available at: https://academic.oup.com/ofid/article/4/suppl_1/S637/4295469.

93. Hadaway L. Short peripheral intravenous catheters and infections. J Infus Nurs 2012;35(4):230–40.

94. Mermel LA. Short-term peripheral venous catheter-related bloodstream infections: a systematic review. Clin Infect Dis 2017;65(10):1757–62.

95. Rickard CM, Webster J, Wallis MC, et al. Routine versus clinically indicated replacement of peripheral intravenous catheters: a randomised controlled equivalence trial. Lancet 2012;380(9847):1066–74.

96. Webster J, Osborne S, Rickard CM, et al. Clinically-indicated replacement versus routine replacement of peripheral venous catheters. Cochrane Database Syst Rev 2015;(8):CD007798.

97. Mermel LA, Parenteau S, Tow SM. The risk of midline catheterization in hospitalized patients. A prospective study. Ann Intern Med 1995;123(11):841–4.

98. Centers for Disease Control and Prevention (CDC). Adverse reactions associated with midline catheters–united states, 1992-1995. MMWR Morb Mortal Wkly Rep 1996;45(5):101–3.

99. Adams DZ, Little A, Vinsant C, et al. The midline catheter: a clinical review. J Emerg Med 2016;51(3):252–8.

100. Caparas JV, Hu JP. Safe administration of long-term vancomycin through a novel midline catheter: a response to letter to the editor. J Vasc Access 2016;17(4):e92.

101. Xu T, Kingsley L, DiNucci S, et al. Safety and utilization of peripherally inserted central catheters versus midline catheters at a large academic medical center. Am J Infect Control 2016;44(12):1458–61.

102. Sharp R, Esterman A, McCutcheon H, et al. The safety and efficacy of midlines compared to peripherally inserted central catheters for adult cystic fibrosis patients: a retrospective, observational study. Int J Nurs Stud 2014;51(5):694–702.

103. Maki DG, Kluger DM, Crnich CJ. The risk of bloodstream infection in adults with different intravascular devices: a systematic review of 200 published prospective studies. Mayo Clin Proc 2006;81(9):1159–71.

104. Koh DB, Gowardman JR, Rickard CM, et al. Prospective study of peripheral arterial catheter infection and comparison with concurrently sited central venous catheters. Crit Care Med 2008;36(2):397–402.

105. Lucet JC, Bouadma L, Zahar JR, et al. Infectious risk associated with arterial catheters compared with central venous catheters. Crit Care Med 2010;38(4):1030–5.

106. Safdar N, O'Horo JC, Maki DG. Arterial catheter-related bloodstream infection: incidence, pathogenesis, risk factors and prevention. J Hosp Infect 2013;85(3):189–95.

107. Pirracchio R, Legrand M, Rigon MR, et al. Arterial catheter-related bloodstream infections: results of an 8-year survey in a surgical intensive care unit. Crit Care Med 2011;39(6):1372–6.
108. Esteve F, Pujol M, Perez XL, et al. Bacteremia related with arterial catheter in critically ill patients. J Infect 2011;63(2):139–43.
109. Gowardman JR, Lipman J, Rickard CM. Assessment of peripheral arterial catheters as a source of sepsis in the critically ill: a narrative review. J Hosp Infect 2010;75(1):12–8.
110. Cohen DM, Carino GP, Heffernan DS, et al. Arterial catheter use in the ICU: a national survey of antiseptic technique and perceived infectious risk. Crit Care Med 2015;43(11):2346–53.
111. Nguyen DB, Shugart A, Lines C, et al. National Healthcare Safety Network (NHSN) Dialysis Event Surveillance Report for 2014. Clin JAm Soc Nephrol 2017;12:1–8.
112. Levin A, Mason AJ, Jindal KK, et al. Prevention of hemodialysis subclavian vein catheter infections by topical povidone-iodine. Kidney Int 1991;40(5):934–8.
113. Lok CE, Stanley KE, Hux JE, et al. Hemodialysis infection prevention with polysporin ointment. J Am Soc Nephrol 2003;14(1):169–79.
114. Hemmelgarn BR, Moist LM, Lok CE, et al. Prevention of dialysis catheter malfunction with recombinant tissue plasminogen activator. N Engl J Med 2011; 364(4):303–12.

Vascular Graft Infections
An update

Amal Gharamti, MD[a], Zeina A. Kanafani, MD, MS, CIC[a,b],*

KEYWORDS

- Vascular graft infection • Vascular reconstructive surgery • Biofilm • Bacteremia
- Staphylococci

KEY POINTS

- Vascular graft infections can be divided into intracavitary, located within the abdomen and thorax, and extracavitary grafts, located in the groin.
- Vascular graft infections occur either in the immediate postoperative period, mainly because of contamination during the procedure, or later, due to graft seeding following bacteremia.
- The most common Gram-positive organisms implicated in vascular graft infections are coagulase-negative staphylococci, followed by methicillin-sensitive Staphylococcus aureus. The most common Gram-negative organism is Pseudomonas aeruginosa.
- Patient-specific risk factors include periodontal disease, nasal colonization with S aureus, postoperative bacteremia and graft characteristics, and diabetes mellitus and postoperative hyperglycemia. Procedure-specific risk factors include incision in the groin area, wound infection, and emergency procedure.
- Initial antibiotic therapy requires broad Gram-positive and Gram-negative coverage. Rifampin-based combinations are preferable, owing to its anti-biofilm activity. Antibiotic therapy, combined with surgical intervention, is associated with better outcomes compared to antibiotic therapy alone.

INTRODUCTION

The early 1950s witnessed the introduction of vascular reconstruction surgery using prosthetic vascular grafts.[1] These grafts are important in the management of peripheral artery disease, arterial aneurysms, and in the establishment of an arteriovenous access for hemodialysis.[2] The use of vascular grafts has led to a significant improvement in the quality of life in patients with vascular disease.[3] The increase in the use of

[a] Division of Infectious Diseases, Department of Internal Medicine, American University of Beirut, Cairo Street, Riad El Solh, Beirut 1107 2020, Lebanon; [b] Division of Infectious Diseases, Department of Internal Medicine, American University of Beirut Medical Center, Cairo Street, PO Box 11-0236/11D, Riad El Solh, Beirut 1107 2020, Lebanon
* Corresponding author. American University of Beirut Medical Center, Cairo Street, PO Box 11-0236/11D, Riad El Solh, Beirut 1107 2020, Lebanon.
E-mail address: zk10@aub.edu.lb

Infect Dis Clin N Am 32 (2018) 789–809
https://doi.org/10.1016/j.idc.2018.06.003
0891-5520/18/© 2018 Elsevier Inc. All rights reserved.
id.theclinics.com

vascular reconstructive surgery has been accompanied with a concomitant increase in the incidence of vascular graft infections (VGIs). VGI is a rare, yet grave complication of vascular surgery.[1] Infections are associated with a high mortality rate, a high amputation rate of affected extremities, and a possibility of reinfection.[4–6] Vascular grafts can be divided into 2 categories: extracavitary, located in the groin, and intracavitary, located in the abdomen and thorax.[1] The incidence of intracavitary aortic graft infections is 0.2% to 5.0%[1,7–9] and the incidence of extracavitary graft infections can be as high as 6%.[1,10] Intracavitary aortic graft infections have a higher mortality (24%–75%) compared with extracavitary graft infections (17%). However, extracavitary graft infections are associated with high morbidity, with an amputation rate of up to 40%.[3]

In this review, we provide a summary of the available data regarding the pathogenesis, microbiology, and mechanisms of invasiveness in VGI. We also address the risk factors that predispose to such infections as well as the clinical manifestations and the available diagnostic techniques. Finally, we comment on the treatment strategies and prevention of VGI.

PATHOGENESIS

Studies have demonstrated 2 peaks in the incidence of VGIs after graft implantation. The first peak occurs in the early postoperative period and is largely due to contamination at the time of surgery or by direct extension from a superficial infection to the graft. The second peak occurs after a long time from the index surgery and is thought to be due to seeding of the graft by a new bacteremia or activation of a dormant infection.[3,11] Graft infections are, therefore, thought to arise as a result of either contamination at the time of graft insertion or a hematogenous infection.[12,13] Contamination during surgery may occur owing to the use of a nonsterile graft, inadequate sterile techniques, contact with the patient's skin or intraabdominal organs, or deposition of airborne particles into the surgical bed. Contamination from the skin of the groin is the most frequent cause of graft infection. The groin incision may cut through infected lymphatic channels or glands, owing to distal infected tissues or ulcers, resulting in direct graft contamination. In addition, the groin incision cuts through skin creases and has a tendency to gape. In obese patients, the surgical wound lies within moist skin folds.[13,14] The vascular graft remains susceptible to infection up to 1 year after implantation, as long as the pseudointimal lining is not yet well-developed. Thereafter, bacteremia can secondarily contaminate the vascular graft.[15] When vascular grafts are infected, the infection will likely spread to native vessels, resulting in inflammation and subsequent disruption of the graft–artery anastomosis and erosion, leading to hemorrhage or the formation of a false aneurysm.[13]

MICROBIOLOGY

Staphylococcus aureus used to be the most frequently isolated organism in infected vascular grafts. More recently, coagulase-negative staphylococci have been recognized as the most common cause of VGI.[1,16] In a retrospective cohort study involving 478 patients undergoing prosthetic bypass grafts of the femoral artery, *Staphylococcus epidermidis* was recovered from 37% of infected grafts, followed by methicillin-sensitive *S aureus* (26%), enterococci (10%), methicillin-resistant *S aureus* (MRSA), *Pseudomonas* species, and others.[10] *Pseudomonas* species are the most common gram-negative bacilli responsible for VGI.[1] In general, gram-negative pathogens are recovered in the setting of an aortoenteric fistula.[3] Other organisms implicated in VGI include anaerobes, fungi,[17] *Cutibacterium* (formerly *Propionibacterium*) species,[18] and other gram-negative organisms such as *Klebsiella pneumoniae*,[10] *Prevotella* species, and

Salmonella species.[7] *Pasteurella multocida* has also been reported and should be suspected as the cause of VGI in patients with or animal scratches or bites.[19,20]

Many factors contribute to this microbiological epidemiology, such as the use of prophylactic antistaphylococcal antibiotics, the improvement in surgical techniques, performing surgery on patients with multiple underlying comorbidities, evolution of the hospital flora, and many others.[1,14] The microbiology of VGIs is also influenced by the location of the graft. In one study,[21] staphylococci were more likely to be isolated from thoracic and peripheral VGIs, whereas abdominal VGIs were polymicrobial, growing gram-negative bacteria, anaerobes, enterococci, and *Candida* species (**Box 1**).

MECHANISMS OF INVASIVENESS
Biofilm Production

Staphylococci are capable of establishing infection through biofilm formation.[16,22] Staphylococcal biofilm formation can be divided into 3 phases: attachment, maturation, and detachment (**Fig. 1**). During the first phase, surface proteins mediate the initial attachment to host matrix proteins such as fibrinogen and fibronectin. Then in the maturation phase, intercellular aggregation, mediated by polysaccharide intercellular adhesin, and biofilm structuring take place. Finally, single cells or clusters of cells detach from the biofilm, resulting in the dissemination of infection.[22]

Biofilms provide resistance to antibiotics mainly by preventing them from reaching the bacterial cells in the biofilm matrix and by limiting their efficacy.[22–24] In addition to their antibiotic resistance, biofilms protect the bacteria against the innate immune system. By shielding the cells within the matrix, neutrophils are prevented from reaching them for phagocytosis.[22,25,26]

Virulence Factors

α-Toxin of S aureus

α-Toxin, also called α-hemolysin, is a common virulence factor of *S aureus* pathogenic strains. It is initially secreted as a water-soluble monomer, capable of oligomerization on the host cell membrane, resulting in pore formation and cellular lysis.[27,28] Caiazza and O'Toole[29] proposed that α-hemolysin plays a role in biofilm formation, by mediating cell–cell interaction. They showed that mutant strains, carrying a mutant α-hemolysin gene, are capable of colonizing a surface, but would not fulfill the maturation phase and form colonies. ADAM10, a zinc-dependent metalloprotease, has been shown to function as a cellular receptor for α-toxin. Inoshima and colleagues[30] showed that mice lacking the ADAM10 receptor in the respiratory epithelium had a marked improvement in the outcome of pneumonia caused by both methicillin-sensitive *S aureus* and MRSA.

Box 1
Organisms commonly implicated in vascular graft infections

Coagulase-negative staphylococci (most common)

Methicillin-sensitive *S aureus*

Methicillin-resistant *S aureus*

Pseudomonas species (most common among gram-negative organisms)

Anaerobes

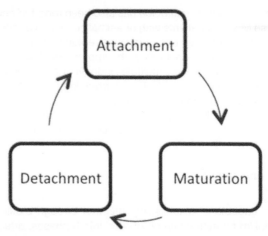

Fig. 1. Phases of biofilm development.

Cell wall–anchored proteins

S aureus expresses on its surface an abundance of cell wall-anchored (CWA) proteins that facilitate the bacteria's adhesion and invasion into host tissues. These CWA proteins include fibronectin-binding protein A, collagen-binding protein, protein A, clumping factor A, and clumping factor B, each with a specific function. For example, fibronectin-binding proteins promote the adhesion and internalization of *S aureus* into host cells, and protein A impairs opsonization allowing *S aureus* to escape opsonophagocytosis.[31,32] *S epidermidis* expresses CWA proteins that mediate infection in humans, but to a lesser extent than *S aureus*.[33]

RISK FACTORS
Patient-Specific Risk Factors

Periodontal disease

Thomas and colleagues[34] described a possible association between periodontal disease and late-onset VGIs. They reported 4 cases of VGIs, three of which had 16S ribosomal DNA gene analysis, confirming that the bacterial mixture causing the infection was oral in origin. Furthermore, all 3 cases had severe periodontal disease, confirmed postoperatively after the results of nucleic acid amplification. Therefore, the authors suggest that periodontal disease could be a risk factor for late-onset prosthetic VGIs, acknowledging the need for more studies on this matter. A systematic review of 44 studies[35] found that there was a general agreement on the need to screen and treat dental infections before cardiovascular procedures; however, protocols were lacking.

Nasal colonization with S aureus

Nasal colonization with *S aureus* has been shown in many studies to increase the risk of vascular surgical site infections.[36] In fact, nasal carriers of a high burden of *S aureus* are 3 to 6 times more likely to develop a health care–associated infection compared with noncarriers or carriers of a lower burden.[37,38] Safdar and Bradley[39] showed that MRSA colonization poses a 4-fold increased risk of clinical infection compared with methicillin-sensitive *S aureus*. In addition, MRSA infection complicating vascular surgery results in significant morbidity, increased hospital duration of stay, and is more likely to result in amputation and graft removal.[40] The mechanism by which *S aureus* nasal colonization is thought to result in postoperative infections is by direct transmission from the nares to the surgical site via the patient's hands.[41]

Postoperative bacteremia and graft characteristics

Moore and colleagues[42] showed that the aortic grafts, before the formation of a pseudointima, are susceptible to infection in the setting of transient bacteremia. In another study, bacteremia was associated with a higher risk of developing aortic graft infections.[6] Rosenman and colleagues[43] investigated the different susceptibility of commonly used grafts to S aureus adherence. Using indium-111 and a pulsatile perfusion system, they found that polytetrafluoroethylene (PTFE) grafts were the least likely to harbor bacteria, with umbilical vein grafts harboring 5 times more bacteria and Dacron grafts 50 times more. In addition, the presence of a suture line in PTFE grafts increased their susceptibility to bacterial adherence. This difference in bacterial adherence is attributed to the different graft characteristics, such as graft fiber surface characteristics, the material's hydrophobicity, and the surface charge of the graft. Different bacteria and different strains within the same bacterial species have different adherence capacities. Using ultrasonic oscillation, Schmitt and colleagues[44] studied the adherence capability of different bacteria (S aureus, non–mucin-producing S epidermidis, mucin-producing S epidermidis, and Escherichia coli) to expanded PTFE (ePTFE), woven Dacron, and velour knitted Dacron. All bacterial strains had the greatest affinity to velour knitted Dacron. The purpose of the addition of velour to Dacron grafts is to enhance the graft's attachment to the perigraft tissue, resulting in improved development of an intimal lining, proven previously to decrease the risk of infection after bacteremia. However, the increased bacterial adherence to velour knitted Dacron grafts is probably related to the porous nature of the graft, providing greater surface area for bacterial adherence. Another important observation in this study was that the production of mucin by mucin-producing S epidermidis strains significantly increased bacterial adherence to both ePTFE and velour knitted Dacron compared with S aureus and non–mucin-producing S epidermidis.

Diabetes mellitus and postoperative hyperglycemia

Vriesendorp and colleagues[45] showed that postoperative hyperglycemia was associated with a higher risk of postoperative infections in vascular surgery, although the risk was decreased in patients with diabetes. They attributed these results to the use of insulin in diabetic patients and its absence in nondiabetics but who have postoperative hyperglycemia. Insulin has been shown to have antiinflammatory effect in both humans and animal experiments whereas glucose has been shown to have a proinflammatory effect.[46] Other studies consistently reported diabetes to be a risk factor for VGIs.[10,16,47] This finding can be attributed to the impaired immune response observed in patients with diabetes.[48]

Procedure-Specific Risk Factors

Location of the incision

Groin incision has been shown in many studies to be a significant risk factor for VGIs.[16,41,49] The groin area is particularly susceptible to infections because of its rich microbial flora,[49] the proximity of this area to the perineum, and the superficial location of vascular grafts in the groin.[50]

Wound infection

This entity poses an added risk for VGI possibly by direct extension.[10,49]

Emergency procedure

It has been shown that emergency procedures are associated with an increased risk for prosthetic VGIs.[3,16,41] This is due to insufficient time, resulting in inadequate patient preparation before surgery and, thus, a greater risk for contamination and subsequent VGI.[14]

Additional risk factors for VGI include inappropriate antibiotic prophylaxis, invasive procedures before or after graft placement, poor wound healing, comorbid conditions like chronic renal insufficiency and an immunocompromised state, prolonged operation time, and prolonged duration of hospital stay before the index surgery.[3,41]

CLINICAL CLASSIFICATION

Szilagyi and colleagues[12] classified VGIs into grades I, II, and III infections. Grade I infections are the most superficial, and they involve the dermis only; grade II infections extend beyond the dermis into the subcutaneous tissue but do not reach the vascular implant; and when the implant is affected, the infection is classified as grade III. Whereas grades I and II infections are usually easy to manage, grade III infections pose the greatest therapeutic challenge. Another classification system by Bunt[51] divides infections into graft infections, graft–enteric erosions, graft–enteric fistulae, and aortic stump sepsis. Noticing different microorganisms as the cause of infection in early and late infections, Bandyk[52] classified graft infections according to the organisms implicated. Finally, Samson and colleagues[53] divided VGIs into 5 groups, depending on the extent of infection and the structures involved (**Table 1**).

CLINICAL MANIFESTATIONS

Early VGIs occur within the first 4 months after graft placement surgery, whereas late VGIs occur after 4 months. However, early VGIs mostly occur within the first 2 months postoperatively.[21] Early VGIs are usually caused by virulent bacteria, such as *S aureus,* and gram-negative bacteria, such as *E coli, Proteus* species, and *P aeruginosa.* Late infections are usually caused by less virulent bacteria such as *S epidermidis.*

Early infections are usually easier to diagnose, because the signs and symptoms of infection and inflammation are more apparent. Patients may present with signs of sepsis such as fever, chills, and leukocytosis. Other findings include sinus tract drainage, abscess, limb ischemia as a result of thrombotic occlusion of the infected graft, and local signs such as erythema and tenderness of the skin overlying the graft. Late-onset infections are usually indolent, with signs of systemic sepsis often lacking.[1,16] Patients with abdominal VGIs can present with an aortoenteric fistula, whereas patients with thoracic VGIs can present with an aortobronchial fistula.[21]

Table 1	
Samson classification of vascular graft infections	
Group	**Areas of Involvement**
I	Dermis only
II	Subcutaneous tissue but not the graft
III	Body of the graft without the anastomosis
IV	Graft and anastomosis, without bacteremia or anastomotic bleeding
V	Graft and anastomosis, with bacteremia and/or anastomotic bleeding

DIAGNOSIS

The approach to the patient presenting with a suspected VGI starts with obtaining an accurate medical history and performing a thorough physical examination. Leukocytosis and increased inflammatory markers, such as C-reactive protein, are seen commonly. A Gram stain and culture should be taken for blood and any wound before antibiotic administration.[5]

Extracavitary Infections

According to the American Heart Association, the initial imaging modality of choice when suspecting a VGI is ultrasound examination.[1] It is widely available, inexpensive, quick, and poses no risk of kidney injury, because it does not need contrast material for visualization. Ultrasound examination allows evaluation for pseudoaneurysm formation or any fluid collection. When ultrasound examination findings are indeterminate, computed tomography (CT) angiography or MRI can be considered. When these 2 modalities also prove to be unhelpful in confirming a diagnosis of VGI, a PET/CT scan or indium-labeled white blood cell study scan can be done. PET/CT is useful in the setting of late infections, where the symptoms are nonspecific and nonlocalizing, and where all other diagnostic modalities have provided no evidence of a focus of infection.[54] In a prospective cohort study involving 34 patients suspected to have a VGI, Sah and colleagues[55] aimed at investigating the diagnostic accuracy of PET/CT with fludeoxyglucose F 18 in VGIs. The sensitivity, specificity, positive predictive value, negative predictive value, and accuracy of FDG-PET/CT were 100%, 86%, 96%, 100%, and 97%, respectively. Therefore, PET/CT scanning is an effective diagnostic tool in VGIs.

Intracavitary Infections

It is recommended to perform a CT angiography scan as the initial imaging modality. If the CT angiography scan does not provide a diagnosis and the suspicion of a VGI is high, an MRI, PET/CT, or indium white blood cell study scan can be considered. In the setting of an aortoenteric fistula and gastrointestinal bleeding, patients should undergo esophagogastroduodenoscopy to look for erosions, ulcers, or thrombi. When the infected vascular graft is intrathoracic, imaging findings should be combined with blood culture results and echocardiography.[1]

MANAGEMENT

Determining the best management plan for an infected vascular graft depends on the location of the graft, the extent of the infection, and the organism(s) implicated.[14] The optimal management of prosthetic VGIs involves excision of the graft, complete debridement of the infected surrounding tissues, restoration of blood flow distal to the infected graft, and, finally, appropriate antibiotic therapy.[3]

Antibiotic Therapy

Empiric antibiotic therapy should be parenterally administered, with targeted activity against the organisms expected to grow in culture. In addition, the antibiotic should have an antibiofilm activity enabling it to penetrate into the biofilm and kill slow-growing bacteria. Once the antibiotic susceptibilities become available, antibiotic therapy can be adjusted or deescalated to cover the implicated organism(s). Initial therapy involves broad gram-positive coverage (accounting for MRSA), and broad gram-negative coverage (accounting for *Pseudomonas*). Daptomycin, vancomycin, or linezolid can be used for gram-positive coverage and the antipseudomonal β-lactams can be used for initial gram-negative coverage.[2] In patients with penicillin allergy, fluoroquinolones can substitute for β-lactams.[56]

Daptomycin is the preferred antibiotic. Vancomycin and linezolid are active against MRSA; however, unlike daptomycin, they demonstrate time-dependent slowly bactericidal or bacteriostatic activity and lack antibiofilm activity.[56] Daptomycin is a cyclic lipopeptide exhibiting rapid concentration-dependent bactericidal activity against staphylococci, enterococci, and streptococci. It has been approved for the treatment of complicated skin and soft tissue infections, right-sided endocarditis, and MRSA bacteremia.[57] In an in vitro study using a guinea pig foreign body infection model, the use of a combination of high-dose daptomycin (>6 mg/kg) and rifampin was associated with greater killing of planktonic and adherent MRSA.[58] In addition, Legout and colleagues[59] showed in a retrospective study of 26 patients treated for prosthetic VGI that the use of high-dose daptomycin (>8 mg/kg) is a potentially successful approach with acceptable side effects in the severely ill patient population.

Conservative treatment with antibiotic therapy alone, without surgical intervention, is associated with high mortality.[60] However, in a study conducted by Erb and colleagues,[21] among 17.6% of the patients who were treated conservatively, the cure rate exceeded 90%. The management should be highly individualized, with the choice of conservative treatment reserved for a limited carefully selected group.[60] In the same study by Erb and colleagues,[21] treatment with a rifampicin-based regimen was associated with a higher cure rate. Similarly, another study showed that the nonuse of rifampin in the treatment of prosthetic VGIs was associated with poor outcome.[61] It was, therefore, suggested that rifampin-based combinations be used as definite therapy to achieve a better response. The use of combination therapy aims at preventing the emergence of bacterial resistance. In an in vitro study conducted by Cirioni and colleagues,[62] the use of both daptomycin and rifampin had a greater efficacy against S aureus infections compared with the use of either antibiotic alone. In addition, the use of rifampin alone resulted in the emergence of 4 resistant isolates, although no resistance was observed when daptomycin was administered concomitantly with rifampin.

There are no clinical trials that have evaluated the optimal duration of antibiotic therapy after a VGI. However, there is general consensus that at least 4 to 6 weeks of parenteral antibiotic therapy is necessary. In cases of partial graft excision or graft preservation, patients may be placed on lifelong suppressive therapy.[2,63]

Surgical Management

Surgical excision with extraanatomic bypass

Aggressive management of prosthetic VGIs, including excision of the graft, debridement of infected tissues, and extraanatomic bypass if collateral circulation is inadequate, has been the standard of care.[64] To avoid prolonged tissue ischemia distally, it is essential to construct the extraanatomic bypass first through noninfected tissue and then remove the infected graft.[63,65] O'Hara and colleagues[66] reported that patients undergoing a staged procedure experienced a significantly lower amputation rate (7%) compared with the group of patients in which graft excision and the extraanatomic bypass were performed in a combined procedure (41%; $P = .04$). Also, in a retrospective review of aortic graft infection cases, the best results were seen when the standard approach is taken.[65] After a follow-up period of 34 months, none of the patients undergoing total excision with extraanatomic bypass experienced complications of recurrent infection or amputation. Finally, in a case series of 36 patients treated for aortic graft infection with extraanatomic bypass and graft removal, the postoperative mortality rate was 11% and the overall treatment-related mortality was 19.4%.[4] Four patients (11%) eventually required amputations in the postoperative period. The 5-year survival was 56%, and recurrent infection occurred in only 1 patient with bilateral axillofemoral bypass graft infection.

The high morbidity and mortality associated with the aforementioned approach has led to the consideration of alternative options, such as excision and in situ replacement of the infected graft.[64] The study conducted by Erb and colleagues[21] showed that graft retention or graft replacement were not associated with treatment failure. The in situ replacement can be done using either prosthetic grafts impregnated with silver or rifampin, to decrease the risk of reinfection, or tissue grafts such as arterial allografts, venous allografts, and venous autografts. Patients with low-grade infections in whom blood and perigraft fluid cultures are negative can benefit from graft resection and in situ replacement, whereas patients with more severe infections in whom blood and perigraft fluid cultures are positive would not, owing to the high mortality rate.[67] There are specific conditions that eliminate any possibility of graft replacement or preservation and necessitate an aggressive management and these include sepsis, anastomotic disruption, aortoenteric fistula, and the presence of virulent organisms like MRSA or *Pseudomonas*. Despite this finding, some patients who are severely ill with many comorbidities are considered high risk and may not qualify for extensive procedures with total graft excision.[63]

In situ reconstruction using antibiotic-impregnated prosthetic grafts

The use of rifampin-soaked grafts has proven appealing owing to its potential in both prevention and treatment of VGIs. Rifampin has activity against staphylococci and a variety of gram-negative pathogens. Torsello and colleagues[68] reported 5 cases in which the gold standard of management was not feasible. Therefore, they resorted to the use of rifampin-soaked grafts. There was no recurrence of infection or any other complication at a follow-up period of 6 months to 1 year. Another study showed that total graft excision followed by the in situ placement of a rifampin-soaked grafts is a feasible option with favorable long-term results[69]; however, it can be limited in the setting of an MRSA infection. Bandyk and colleagues[64] recommended the use of rifampin-soaked prosthetic grafts for in situ treatment of VGIs in a selective patient population. They showed that it can be safely used in patients with low-grade gram-positive infections and that failure of this technique was due to infections caused by virulent and resistant strains. Having in mind that the use of rifampin as a single agent can result in the emergence of resistance, Aboshady and colleagues[70] investigated the effectiveness of Dacron grafts bonded with rifampin, minocycline, and chlorhexidine in resisting colonization and infection during the first 8 weeks postoperatively in a pig model. Before implantation, the triple antibiotic-bonded grafts were immersed into an *S aureus* solution. Eight weeks after implantation, there was no bacterial growth detected on the grafts.

Some patients with VGI present in such a debilitated condition that they do not qualify for open repair. These patients are managed with endografts. Escobar and colleagues[71] reported the case of a 66-year-old patient with a history of aortic patch angioplasty presenting with hemorrhagic shock owing to an aortoduodenal fistula. The patient was managed with a rifampin-soaked endograft without removing the infected graft or repairing the duodenum. This process allowed the immediate management of her life-threatening condition, delaying the definitive procedure so it could be done electively at a later stage when the patient would be in a stable condition. Until now, there are no clinical trials to evaluate the use of rifampin-soaked grafts in the treatment of VGIs compared with non–antibiotic-impregnated grafts in terms of reinfection rates and other outcomes. It is worth mentioning that Schneider and colleagues[72] previously showed in a dog model areas of necrosis at the anastomotic sites of the rifampin-soaked graft, with no evidence of bacterial colonization and suggested that this finding might be due to rifampin toxicity. In light of the potential for toxicity, the use of rifampin-soaked grafts should be reassessed and studied carefully.

In contrast, endolysins, which are bacteriophage-based enzymes aiming at destroying the peptidoglycan layer of bacteria, have become interesting candidates in lieu of traditional antimicrobial agents.[73] In addition, in light of their low toxicity,[72] their potential use for impregnating grafts before their placement in the human body should be explored.

In situ reconstruction using cryopreserved arterial allografts

The use of biological grafts such as autologous veins and human allografts may provide increased resistance to infection compared with prosthetic grafts. They can be implanted inside an infected surgical field after resection of the infected graft.[74] This increased resistance has not been affirmed, but it could be related to the better antibiotic diffusion and attraction of immune cells into the allograft wall.[75] Excellent results had been obtained previously with the treatment of endocarditis with cryopreserved allograft valves.[76] This finding has led to the use of allografts in the settings of VGIs. The use of fresh allografts has been abandoned owing to the high associated complication rate.[77] Vogt and colleagues[78] compared the use of cryopreserved arterial allograft with prosthetic material in the management of mycotic aneurysms or prosthetic VGIs. The use of cryopreserved arterial allografts was associated with better disease-related survival, disease-related survival free of reoperation, duration of intensive care, duration of postoperative antibiotic therapy, incidence of complications, elimination of infection, and costs. In a large published case series evaluating the use of 220 cryopreserved allografts in patients with aortic graft infections,[79] the authors recommended the use of arterial allografts as a first-line treatment for aortic graft infections. Despite the effectiveness of cryopreserved arterial allografts in the management of prosthetic VGIs, the complications reported in the literature include allograft thrombosis, anastomotic pseudoaneurysm, aneurysmal degeneration, and allograft disruption.[80,81] A high 5-year reintervention rate has been reported for patients with prosthetic VGIs treated with cryopreserved allografts, reaching 55% when the intervention is at the aortoiliac level and 33% at the peripheral level.[81] Lowampa and colleagues[80] proposed several interventions to minimize allograft-related complications. The authors proposed avoiding size mismatch when using several allografts for aortic reconstruction and using through-and-through transfixing polypropylene stitches in ligating the collateral side branches of the allograft. Finally, in the setting of an aortoenteric fistula, the authors recommend wide resection of the bowel harboring the fistula followed by intestinal reanastomosis away from the area of vascular repair. A recent study has evaluated the use of cryopreserved arterial allografts for in situ reconstruction of an abdominal aortic native graft or secondary graft infection.[82] The reintervention rate was 12.7% (9 of 71) for the following complications: proximal anastomotic rupture (n = 1), stenosis/thrombosis (n = 5), ureteral–graft fistula (n = 1), and distal anastomosis false aneurysm (n = 2). Primary patency after 5 years was 93%.

Graft sparing

The treatment of prosthetic thoracic aortic graft infections is associated with significant morbidity and mortality in the range of 25% to 27%.[83,84] Therefore, an aggressive surgical management is not always possible. In a selected patient population, and when the VGI occurs less than 1 month after the index procedure, graft preservation might be an option. Graft-sparing therapy involves aggressive debridement with anti-biotic irrigation and systemic antibiotic therapy for at least 2 weeks.[84] However, when the patient presents with signs of graft infection 3 to 6 months after the index surgery, graft replacement is always preferred. This phenomenon is probably related to the life-cycle of a biofilm. Early in the postoperative period, biofilms are still immature and thus easier to eradicate, whereas in the late postoperative period, biofilms have become mature, making graft preservation an unviable option.[85,86]

Management of complications

Aortoenteric fistula is a serious complication of aortic graft infections.[87] Standard treatment of abdominal VGIs complicated by aortoenteric fistula is a staged proced-ure that consists of an axillofemoral bypass through a noninfected field, graft removal, and closure of the aortic stump.[88] Oderich and colleagues[87] investigated the in situ replacement of the infected grafts complicated with aortoenteric fistula with rifampin-soaked grafts. Their surgical technique consists of excising the infected graft, repairing the intestinal defect, placement of the in situ rifampin-soaked graft, and finally covering the graft with omentum. The patients are then treated with long-term oral antibiotic suppression. This technique could be used in patients with limited infection, but not in those patients with large abscesses and excessive purulence.

Another complication of aortic graft infections is the formation of an aortoesopha-geal fistula, with patients typically presenting with gastrointestinal bleeding. If the pa-tient is hemodynamically unstable on presentation, thoracic endovascular aortic repair can be done as an emergent procedure to stabilize the patient.[89] However, thoracic endovascular aortic repair will not repair the esophageal defect nor control the infec-tion and, therefore, the risk of graft infection and fistula recurrence remains.[90] Before the final surgical management, the patient's general medical condition should be sta-bilized and broad-spectrum antibiotics should be administered. Radical surgery then follows, with debridement and excision of the infected tissue, extraanatomic bypass or in situ repair, and repair of the esophageal defect.[89,90] The optimal duration from thoracic endovascular aortic repair to definitive surgical therapy is usually no longer than 1 week to avoid progression of the infection.[91]

Management of peripheral grafts

As indicated, the incidence of extracavitary graft infections can be as high as 6%.[1] The gravity of peripheral graft infections as compared with aortic graft infections is related to the high rate of morbidity and mortality associated with this complication. The risk of limb loss and amputation can reach 41%.[92] The surgical management of peripheral graft infections is similar to aortic graft infections and it consists of one of the following: complete graft excision with extraanatomic bypass or in situ reconstruction, partial graft excision, or complete retention of the graft.[92–94] Caution should be exercised while selecting patients to undergo partial graft excision or graft preservation as the rate of reinfection and subsequent need for reoperation could be high. Mertens and colleagues[92] reported that 82% of the peripheral graft infection cases managed with partial graft excision required reoperations for sepsis control, compared with only 13% of the cases managed with total graft excision. Therefore, total graft removal is the preferred management strategy for patients presenting with peripheral graft infections.[95]

Management of infected arteriovenous grafts

In the setting of anastomotic involvement, presence of virulent organisms, or sepsis, complete or total graft excision is advocated. In the absence of any of the former conditions, subtotal graft excision can be considered. In subtotal graft excision, a small part of the prosthetic graft is retained, maintaining the arterial lumen patent.[2,96] The incidence of recurrent infection as a complication of subtotal graft excision is conflicting in the literature, with some studies reporting increased incidence of recurrence and others reporting no increased risk of recurrent infection.[96–98] Other surgical approaches involve partial graft excision with bypass in the setting of a localized infection. The advantage of this technique lies in the possibility of immediate cannulation postoperatively for dialysis, thereby eliminating the need to establish a temporary dialysis access. However, similar to subtotal graft excision, partial graft excision carries the risk of a recurrent infection.[96]

In summary, the optimal surgical intervention for prosthetic VGIs remains controversial. The treatment should be highly individualized and depends on the availability of autologous veins, cryopreserved allografts, or prosthetic grafts, as well as the surgeon's experience.[80] **Fig. 2** is a simplified flowchart to aid in the management of VGIs.

PREVENTION

Given the often devastating effects of VGIs, significant efforts have been directed at various preventive strategies. **Table 2** lists some of the risk factors of VGIs and potential preventive methods.

Decolonization

Bode and colleagues[38] conducted a randomized, double-blind, placebo-controlled trial to assess the efficacy of screening for *S aureus* and subsequent decolonization

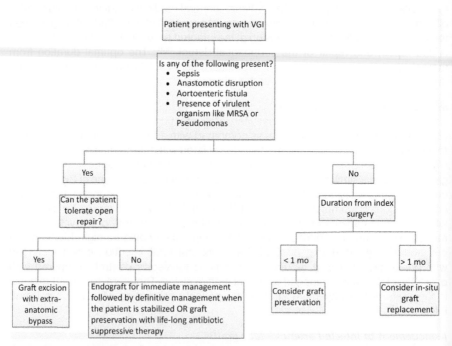

Fig. 2. General management of vascular graft infections (VGIs). MRSA, methicillin-resistant *Staphylococcus aureus*.

Table 2
Risk factors and possible preventive strategies of vascular graft infections

Risk Factors	Prevention	Comments
Colonization with *S aureus*	• Use of mupirocin for nasal decolonization and chlorhexidine for extranasal carriage • Use of vaccines that target *S aureus*	• Mupirocin decolonization carries with it the risk of emergence of resistance, so its use should be reserved for high-risk patients. • Vaccines targeting *S aureus* should be further explored as they eliminate the need for decolonization and the subsequent dilemma of antibiotic resistance.
Extensive dental disease	Screen for and treat dental infections before vascular procedures	• There are no randomized clinical trials to confirm the effectiveness of treating dental infections before vascular procedures. • There are no protocols that make this a preventive strategy and standard practice.
Use of prosthetic grafts (eg, Dacron)	Use of autologous grafts, cryopreserved human allografts, or tissue-engineered vascular grafts	• Tissue-engineered allografts offer the possibility of a nonimmunogenic, nonthrombogenic graft; however, they are still under development.
Intraoperative and postoperative contamination	• Antibiotic prophylaxis within 60 min of the incision • Collagen-implant impregnated with gentamicin sulfate • Negative pressure wound therapy • Use of antibiotic- or endolysin-impregnated vascular grafts	• More research is needed to prove the superiority of negative pressure wound therapy to standard occlusive dressings. • The toxicity of antibiotics in antibiotic-impregnated grafts might limit their future use, and the use of endolysin-impregnated grafts should be further studied.
Diabetes mellitus and postoperative hyperglycemia	Tight sugar control in patients undergoing vascular procedures	• Diabetes results in an impaired immune response. • Insulin has been shown to have antiinflammatory effects.

in the prevention of surgical site infections. A total of 917 patients with positive nasal swabs for *S aureus* on admission were divided into treatment group (504 patients), receiving mupirocin and chlorhexidine, and into placebo group (413 patients). In the treatment group, 3.4% of patients developed *S aureus* infections compared with 7.7% in the placebo group. This trial proved that the use of both mupirocin (for nasal carriage) and chlorhexidine (for extranasal carriage) resulted in a significant decrease in surgical site infections. However, caution should be exercised if hospitals decide to implement this preventive strategy. The use of mupirocin can lead to the development of resistance among *S aureus* strains. Therefore, the use of mupirocin should be limited to carriers who are at high risk for infection. Second, to avoid unnecessary use of mupirocin, tests that detect S aureus should be highly specific. A similar trial is needed to assess whether such an intervention could decrease prosthetic VGIs after vascular surgery in particular. In addition to these antimicrobial strategies, nonantimicrobial strategies for the decolonization of S aureus and prevention of S aureus infections have also been investigated. Vaccines that target clumping factor B[99] and alpha-hemolysin[100] are still under experimentation and may prove to be effective for S aureus decolonization and prevention of S aureus infections.

Tissue-Engineered Vascular Grafts

Birinyi and colleagues[11] showed that the presence of an endothelial lining on the surface of vascular grafts is associated with increased resistance to bacterial adherence in dogs. ePTFE grafts are one of the most commonly used grafts in vascular reconstructive surgery. However, these grafts do not undergo endothelialization. Chen and colleagues[101] presented a method to allow for the endothelialization of ePTFE grafts, via coating the graft with extracellular matrix and CD34 monoclonal antibodies. CD34 monoclonal antibodies serve as a capturing tool for CD34$^+$ endothelial progenitor cells that can differentiate into mature endothelial cells. The addition of extracellular matrix aims at supporting endothelial growth on the surface of the graft. Tissue-engineered vascular grafts could be a promising tool and a better alternative to the currently used synthetic grafts because of their potential nonthrombogenicity and nonimmunogenicity; however, they are still under development.[96,102]

Antibiotic Prophylaxis

The aim of antibiotic prophylaxis is to achieve serum and tissue concentrations of the antibiotic at a level above the minimum inhibitory concentration for organisms likely to have colonized the surgical site to prevent surgical site infections.[103] For vascular procedures, the recommended prophylactic antibiotics are cefazolin and cefuroxime. Antibiotics should be administered within 60 minutes of the incision, and additional dosing is warranted if the surgical procedure persists for more than 2 half-lives of the antibiotic administered (2–5 hours for cefazolin and 3–4 hours for cefuroxime). Antibiotic prophylaxis should be discontinued within 24 hours of the end of surgery, because prolonged prophylaxis duration does not decrease the risk of postoperative infections and has been associated with increased resistance should a surgical site infection occur.[104] In patients allergic to β-lactams, it is recommended to give either vancomycin or clindamycin.[103] With vancomycin use, the infusion should begin 120 minutes before the incision and an additional dose is recommended after 6 to 12 hours for prolonged surgery. With clindamycin, a second dose is needed after 3 to 6 hours.

Some guidelines and observational studies recommend the administration of antibiotic prophylaxis closer to the incision time, within 30 minutes.[105,106] To settle the debate about the optimal timing for administering prophylactic antimicrobial agents, Weber and colleagues[107] conducted a phase III clinical trial that included patients undergoing general, trauma, and vascular surgery. They compared the early administration of antibiotic prophylaxis (within 60 minutes of incision) with late administration (inside the operating room) and did not find any significant difference in the surgical site infection rates between the 2 groups. Therefore, the findings of this trial do not support late administration of antibiotic prophylaxis, and that the dosing within 60 minutes of the incision remains adequate.

Collagen Implant Impregnated with Gentamicin Sulfate (Collatamp)

This implant has been shown to decrease the incidence of surgical site infections in general, cardiac, and orthopedic surgery.[108,109] Almeida and colleagues[110] investigated the usefulness of this implant in the prevention of VGIs. They recruited 60 patients with lower limb ischemia to undergo femoropopliteal PTFE prosthetic bypass and divided them into a control group and an implant group. The control group, in which Collatamp was not used, had a surgical site infection rate of 20% (6 of 30), whereas the implant group, which had Collatamp applied next to the prosthesis, had a surgical site infection rate of 0% (0 of 30). The infections in the control group were grades I and II according to the Szilagyi classification. Because VGIs can develop by direct extension,[10,111] the prevention of a grade I or II infection will likely prevent the occurrence of VGI.[110] A randomized, controlled trial is needed to confirm the validity of these results.

Postoperative Wound Care

As indicated, it is hypothesized that one way by which graft infections develop is by direct extension from a nearby infection, such as a superficial wound infection. Hence, by preventing postoperative wound infection, subsequent graft infection could be prevented as well. Efforts are therefore tailored at creating an optimal sterile environment to promote wound healing. One means by which this can be achieved is via the use of negative pressure wound therapy. Matatov and colleagues[112] investigated the use of Prevena, a new negative pressure incision management system, in the prevention of wound infections in patients undergoing vascular surgery. In the non-Prevena group, the infection rate was 30% (19 of 63) with 10 patients having Szilagyi grade I infections, 7 patients with Szilagyi grade II infections, and 2 patients with Szilagyi grade III infections. In contrast, the infection rate in the Prevena group was significantly lower (6% [3 of 52]; $P = .0011$), with all infections being grade I. In addition, a single-center, randomized, clinical trial was conducted to evaluate the use of negative pressure wound therapy compared with standard dressing in the prevention of postoperative infections after lower extremity vascular surgery in a high-risk population.[113] The postoperative 30-day surgical site infection rate was numerically lower in the negative pressure wound therapy group (11%) compared with the group that received standard dressing (19%); however, the difference was not statistically significant ($P = .24$).

REFERENCES

1. Wilson WR, Bower TC, Creager MA, et al. Vascular graft infections, mycotic aneurysms, and endovascular infections: a scientific statement from the American Heart Association. Circulation 2016;134:e412–60.
2. Young MH, Upchurch GR, Malani PN. Vascular graft infections. Infect Dis Clin North Am 2012;26:41–56.
3. Warner M, Nelson R, Lim C. Vascular graft infection. In: Fitridge R, editor. Oxford textbook of vascular surgery. Oxford University Press; 2016.
4. Seeger JM, Pretus HA, Welborn MB, et al. Long-term outcome after treatment of aortic graft infection with staged extra-anatomic bypass grafting and aortic graft removal. J Vasc Surg 2000;32:451–9 [discussion: 460–1].
5. Mussa FF, Hedayati N, Zhou W, et al. Prevention and treatment of aortic graft infection. Expert Rev Anti Infect Ther 2007;5:305–15.
6. Vogel TR, Symons R, Flum DR. The incidence and factors associated with graft infection after aortic aneurysm repair. J Vasc Surg 2008;47:264–9.

7. Fatima J, Duncan AA, de Grandis E, et al. Treatment strategies and outcomes in patients with infected aortic endografts. J Vasc Surg 2013;58:371–9.

8. Batt M, Feugier P, Camou F, et al. A meta-analysis of outcomes after in situ reconstructions for aortic graft infection. Angiology 2018;69(5):370–9.

9. Berger P, Vaartjes I, Moll FL, et al. Cumulative incidence of graft infection after primary prosthetic aortic reconstruction in the endovascular era. Eur J Vasc Endovasc Surg 2015;49:581–5.

10. Siracuse JJ, Nandivada P, Giles KA, et al. Prosthetic graft infections involving the femoral artery. J Vasc Surg 2013;57:700–5.

11. Birinyi LK, Douville EC, Lewis SA, et al. Increased resistance to bacteremic graft infection after endothelial cell seeding. J Vasc Surg 1987;5:193–7.

12. Szilagyi DE, Smith RF, Elliott JP, et al. Infection in arterial reconstruction with synthetic grafts. Ann Surg 1972;176:321.

13. O'brien T, Collin J. Prosthetic vascular graft infection. Br J Surg 1992;79:1262–7.

14. Chiesa R, Astore D, Frigerio S, et al. Vascular prosthetic graft infection: epidemiology, bacteriology, pathogenesis and treatment. Acta Chir Belg 2002;102: 238–47.

15. Bandyk D. Infection in prosthetic vascular grafts. In: Rutherford RB, editor. Vascular surgery. 6th edition. Philadelphia: Saunders; 2005. p. 875–94.

16. Hicks RC, Greenhalgh RM. The pathogenesis of vascular graft infection. Eur J Vasc Endovasc Surg 1997;14(Suppl A):5–9.

17. Davila VJ, Stone W, Duncan AA, et al. A multicenter experience with the surgical treatment of infected abdominal aortic endografts. J Vasc Surg 2015;62: 877–83.

18. Lyons OT, Patel AS, Saha P, et al. A 14-year experience with aortic endograft infection: management and results. Eur J Vasc Endovasc Surg 2013;46:306–13.

19. Fourreau F, Méchaï F, Brossier J, et al. Vascular graft infection due to Pasteurella multocida. Springerplus 2015;4:824.

20. Kuusela A, Coliondo A, Kourtis A, Vascular graft infection due to Pasteurella multocida. Infection 2004;32:122–3.

21. Erb S, Sidler JA, Elzi L, et al. Surgical and antimicrobial treatment of prosthetic vascular graft infections at different surgical sites: a retrospective study of treatment outcomes. PLoS One 2014;9:e112947.

22. Otto M. Staphylococcal biofilms. Curr Top Microbiol Immunol 2008;322:207–28.

23. Costerton JW, Stewart PS, Greenberg EP. Bacterial biofilms: a common cause of persistent infections. Science 1999;284:1318–22.

24. Keren I, Kaldalu N, Spoering A, et al. Persister cells and tolerance to antimicrobials. FEMS Microbiol Lett 2004;230:13–8.

25. Vuong C, Voyich JM, Fischer ER, et al. Polysaccharide intercellular adhesin (PIA) protects Staphylococcus epidermidis against major components of the human innate immune system. Cell Microbiol 2004;6:269–75.

26. Kocianova S, Vuong C, Yao Y, et al. Key role of poly-gamma-DL-glutamic acid in immune evasion and virulence of Staphylococcus epidermidis. J Clin Invest 2005;115:688–94.

27. Füssle R, Bhakdi S, Sziegoleit A, et al. On the mechanism of membrane damage by Staphylococcus aureus alpha-toxin. J Cell Biol 1981;91:83–94.

28. Bhakdi S, Tranum-Jensen J. Alpha-toxin of Staphylococcus aureus. Microbiol Rev 1991;55:733–51.

29. Caiazza NC, O'toole G. Alpha-toxin is required for biofilm formation by Staphylococcus aureus. J Bacteriol 2003;185:3214–7.

30. Inoshima I, Inoshima N, Wilke GA, et al. A Staphylococcus aureus pore-forming toxin subverts the activity of ADAM10 to cause lethal infection in mice. Nat Med 2011;17:1310–4.
31. Foster TJ, Höök M. Surface protein adhesins of Staphylococcus aureus. Trends Microbiol 1998;6:484–8.
32. Foster TJ, Geoghegan JA, Ganesh VK, et al. Adhesion, invasion and evasion: the many functions of the surface proteins of Staphylococcus aureus. Nat Rev Microbiol 2014;12:49–62.
33. Bowden MG, Chen W, Singvall J, et al. Identification and preliminary characterization of cell-wall-anchored proteins of Staphylococcus epidermidis. Microbiology 2005;151:1453–64.
34. Thomas S, Ghosh J, Porter J, et al. Periodontal disease and late-onset aortic prosthetic vascular graft infection. Case Rep Vasc Med 2015;2015:768935.
35. Cotti E, Arrica M, Di Lenarda A, et al. The perioperative dental screening and management of patients undergoing cardiothoracic, vascular surgery and other cardiovascular invasive procedures: a systematic review. Eur J Prev Cardiol 2017;24:409–25.
36. Bandyk DF. Vascular surgical site infection: risk factors and preventive measures. Semin Vasc Surg 2008;21(3):119–23.
37. Kluytmans JA, Mouton JW, Ijzerman EP, et al. Nasal carriage of Staphylococcus aureus as a major risk factor for wound infections after cardiac surgery. J Infect Dis 1995;171:216–9.
38. Bode LG, Kluytmans JA, Wertheim HF, et al. Preventing surgical-site infections in nasal carriers of Staphylococcus aureus. N Engl J Med 2010;362:9–17.
39. Safdar N, Bradley EA. The risk of infection after nasal colonization with Staphylococcus aureus. Am J Med 2008;121:310–5.
40. Taylor MD, Napolitano LM. Methicillin-resistant Staphylococcus aureus infections in vascular surgery: increasing prevalence. Surg Infect (Larchmt) 2004; 5:180–7.
41. Inui T, Bandyk DF. Vascular surgical site infection: risk factors and preventive measures. Semin Vasc Surg 2015;28:201–7.
42. Moore WS, Rosson CT, Hall AD, et al. Transient bacteremia: a cause of infection in prosthetic vascular grafts. Am J Surg 1969;117:342–3.
43. Rosenman JE, Pearce WH, Kempczinski RF. Bacterial adherence to vascular grafts after in vitro bacteremia. J Surg Res 1985;38:648–55.
44. Schmitt DD, Bandyk DF, Pequet AJ, et al. Bacterial adherence to vascular prostheses: a determinant of graft infectivity. J Vasc Surg 1986;3:732–40.
45. Vriesendorp T, Morelis Q, Devries J, et al. Early post-operative glucose levels are an independent risk factor for infection after peripheral vascular surgery. A retrospective study. Eur J Vasc Endovasc Surg 2004;28:520–5.
46. Dandona P, Chaudhuri A, Ghanim H, et al. Proinflammatory effects of glucose and anti-inflammatory effect of insulin: relevance to cardiovascular disease. Am J Cardiol 2007;99:15–26.
47. Richet H, Chidiac C, Prat A, et al. Analysis of risk factors for surgical wound infections following vascular surgery. Am J Med 1991;91:S170–2.
48. Geerlings SE, Hoepelman AI. Immune dysfunction in patients with diabetes mellitus (DM). Pathog Dis 1999;26:259–65.
49. Antonios VS, Noel AA, Steckelberg JM, et al. Prosthetic vascular graft infection: a risk factor analysis using a case-control study. J Infect 2006;53:49–55.
50. Engin C, Posacioglu H, Ayik F, et al. Management of vascular infection in the groin. Tex Heart Inst J 2005;32:529–34.

51. Bunt T. Synthetic vascular graft infections. I. Graft infections. Surgery 1983;93: 733–46.
52. Bandyk DF. Aortic graft infection. Semin Vasc Surg 1990;3:122–32.
53. Samson RH, Veith FJ, Janko GS, et al. A modified classification and approach to the management of infections involving peripheral arterial prosthetic grafts. J Vasc Surg 1988;8:147–53.
54. Shahani L. Vascular graft infections and role of PET/CT in patients with persistent bacteraemia. BMJ Case Rep 2015;2015 [pii:bcr2014207678].
55. Sah BR, Husmann L, Mayer D, et al. Diagnostic performance of 18F-FDG-PET/CT in vascular graft infections. Eur J Vasc Endovasc Surg 2015;49:455–64.
56. Hodgkiss-Harlow KD, Bandyk DF. Antibiotic therapy of aortic graft infection: treatment and prevention recommendations. Semin Vasc Surg 2011;24:191–8.
57. Kanafani ZA, Corey GR. Daptomycin: a rapidly bactericidal lipopeptide for the treatment of Gram-positive infections. Expert Rev Anti Infec Ther 2007;5: 177–84.
58. John A-K, Baldoni D, Haschke M, et al. Efficacy of daptomycin in implant-associated infection due to methicillin-resistant Staphylococcus aureus: importance of combination with rifampin. Antimicrob Agents Chemother 2009;53: 2719–24.
59. Legout L, D'Elia P, Sarraz-Bournet B, et al. Tolerability of high doses of daptomycin in the treatment of prosthetic vascular graft infection: a retrospective study. Infect Dis Ther 2014;3:215–23.
60. Saleem BR, Meerwaldt R, Tielliu IF, et al. Conservative treatment of vascular prosthetic graft infection is associated with high mortality. Am J Surg 2010; 200:47–52.
61. Legout L, Delia P, Sarraz-Bournet B, et al. Factors predictive of treatment failure in staphylococcal prosthetic vascular graft infections: a prospective observational cohort study: impact of rifampin. BMC Infect Dis 2014;14:228.
62. Cirioni O, Mocchegiani F, Ghiselli R, et al. Daptomycin and rifampin alone and in combination prevent vascular graft biofilm formation and emergence of antibiotic resistance in a subcutaneous rat pouch model of staphylococcal infection. Eur J Vasc Endovasc Surg 2010;40:817–22.
63. Kilic A, Arnaoutakis DJ, Reifsnyder T, et al. Management of infected vascular grafts. Vasc Med 2016;21:53–60.
64. Bandyk DF, Novotney ML, Johnson BL, et al. Use of rifampin-soaked gelatin-sealed polyester grafts for in situ treatment of primary aortic and vascular prosthetic infections. J Surg Res 2001;95:44–9.
65. Ricotta JJ, Faggioli GL, Stella A, et al. Total excision and extra-anatomic bypass for aortic graft infection. Am J Surg 1991;162:145–9.
66. O'Hara PJ, Hertzer NR, Beven EG, et al. Surgical management of infected abdominal aortic grafts: review of a 25-year experience. J Vasc Surg 1986;3: 725–31.
67. Jacobs MJ, Reul GJ, Gregoric I, et al. In-situ replacement and extra-anatomic bypass for the treatment of infected abdominal aortic grafts. Eur J Vasc Surg 1991;5:83–6.
68. Torsello G, Sandmann W, Gehrt A, et al. In situ replacement of infected vascular prostheses with rifampin-soaked vascular grafts: early results. J Vasc Surg 1993;17:768–73.
69. Hayes PD, Nasim A, London NJ, et al. In situ replacement of infected aortic grafts with rifampicin-bonded prostheses: the Leicester experience (1992 to 1998). J Vasc Surg 1999;30:92–8.

70. Aboshady I, Raad I, Vela D, et al. Prevention of perioperative vascular prosthetic infection with a novel triple antimicrobial-bonded arterial graft. J Vasc Surg 2016;64:1805–14.
71. Escobar GA, Eliason JL, Hurie J, et al. Rifampin soaking Dacron-based endografts for implantation in infected aortic aneurysms—new application of a time-tested principle. Ann Vasc Surg 2014;28:744–8.
72. Schneider F, O'Connor S, Becquemin JP. Efficacy of collagen silver-coated polyester and rifampin-soaked vascular grafts to resist infection from MRSA and Escherichia coli in a dog model. Ann Vasc Surg 2008;22:815–21.
73. Schmelcher M, Donovan DM, Loessner MJ. Bacteriophage endolysins as novel antimicrobials. Future Microbiol 2012;7:1147–71.
74. Knosalla C, Goëau-Brissonnière O, Leflon V, et al. Treatment of vascular graft infection by in situ replacement with cryopreserved aortic allografts: an experimental study. J Vasc Surg 1998;27:689–98.
75. Vogt PR, Brunner-LaRocca H-P, Lachat M, et al. Technical details with the use of cryopreserved arterial allografts for aortic infection: influence on early and midterm mortality. J Vasc Surg 2002;35:80–6.
76. McGiffin D, Kirklin J. The impact of aortic valve homografts on the treatment of aortic prosthetic valve endocarditis. Semin Thorac Cardiovasc Surg 1995;7:25–31.
77. Szilagyi DE, Rodriguez FJ, Smith RF, et al. Late fate of arterial allografts: observations 6 to 15 years after implantation. Arch Surg 1970;101:721–33.
78. Vogt PR, Brunner-La Rocca H-P, Carrel T, et al. Cryopreserved arterial allografts in the treatment of major vascular infection: a comparison with conventional surgical techniques. J Thorac Cardiovasc Surg 1998;116:965–72.
79. Harlander-Locke MP, Harmon LK, Lawrence PF, et al. The use of cryopreserved aortoiliac allograft for aortic reconstruction in the United States. J Vasc Surg 2014;59:669–74. e1.
80. Lowampa EM, Holemans C, Stiennon L, et al. Late fate of cryopreserved arterial allografts. Eur J Vasc Endovasc Surg 2016;52:696–702.
81. Lejay A, Delay C, Girsowicz E, et al. Cryopreserved cadaveric arterial allograft for arterial reconstruction in patients with prosthetic infection. Eur J Vasc Endovasc Surg 2017;54(5):636–44.
82. Ahmed SB, Louvancourt A, Daniel G, et al. Cryopreserved arterial allografts for in situ reconstruction of abdominal aortic native or secondary graft infection. J Vasc Surg 2018;67(2):468–77.
83. Takano T, Terasaki T, Wada Y, et al. Treatment of prosthetic graft infection after thoracic aorta replacement. Ann Thorac Cardiovasc Surg 2014;20:304–9.
84. Umminger J, Krueger H, Beckmann E, et al. Management of early graft infections in the ascending aorta and aortic arch: a comparison between graft replacement and graft preservation techniques. Eur J Cardiothorac Surg 2016;50:660–7.
85. Conen A, Fux CA, Vajkoczy P, et al. Management of infections associated with neurosurgical implanted devices. Expert Rev Anti Infect Ther 2017;15:241–55.
86. Gharamti AA, Kanafani ZA. Cutibacterium (formerly Propionibacterium) acnes infections associated with implantable devices. Expert Rev Anti Infect Ther 2017;15(12):1083–94.
87. Oderich GS, Bower TC, Hofer J, et al. In situ rifampin-soaked grafts with omental coverage and antibiotic suppression are durable with low reinfection rates in patients with aortic graft enteric erosion or fistula. J Vasc Surg 2011;53:99–106, 107.e1–7.

88. Reilly LM, Stoney RJ, Goldstone J, et al. Improved management of aortic graft infection: the influence of operation sequence and staging. J Vasc Surg 1987;5: 421–31.

89. Afifi RO, Mushtaq HH, Sandhu HK, et al. Successful multistaged surgical management of secondary aortoesophageal fistula with graft infection. Ann Thorac Surg 2016;101:e203–5.

90. Uno K, Koike T, Takahashi S, et al. Management of aorto-esophageal fistula secondary after thoracic endovascular aortic repair: a review of literature. Clin J Gastroenterol 2017;10:393–402.

91. Okita Y, Yamanaka K, Okada K, et al. Strategies for the treatment of aorto-oesophageal fistula. Eur J Cardiothorac Surg 2014;46:894–900.

92. Mertens RA, O'Hara PJ, Hertzer NR, et al. Surgical management of infrainguinal arterial prosthetic graft infections: review of a thirty-five-year experience. J Vasc Surg 1995;21:782–91.

93. Taylor SM, Weatherford DA, Langan EM, et al. Outcomes in the management of vascular prosthetic graft infections confined to the groin: a reappraisal. Ann Vasc Surg 1996;10:117–22.

94. Calligaro KD, Veith FJ, Dougherty MJ, et al. Management and outcome of infrapopliteal arterial graft infections with distal graft involvement. Am J Surg 1996; 172:178–80.

95. Yeager RA, McConnell DB, Sasaki TM, et al. Aortic and peripheral prosthetic graft infection: differential management and causes of mortality. Am J Surg 1985;150:36–43.

96. Benrashid E, Youngwirth LM, Mureebe L, et al. Operative and perioperative management of infected arteriovenous grafts. J Vasc access 2017;18:13–21.

97. Schild AF, Simon S, Prieto J, et al. Single-center review of infections associated with 1,574 consecutive vascular access procedures. Vasc Endovascular Surg 2003;37:27–31.

98. Walz P, Ladowski JS. Partial excision of infected fistula results in increased patency at the cost of increased risk of recurrent infection. Ann Vasc Surg 2005;19:84–9.

99. Schaffer AC, Solinga RM, Cocchiaro J, et al. Immunization with Staphylococcus aureus clumping factor B, a major determinant in nasal carriage, reduces nasal colonization in a murine model. Infect Immun 2006;74:2145–53.

100. Adhikari RP, Thompson CD, Aman MJ, et al. Protective efficacy of a novel alpha hemolysin subunit vaccine (AT62) against Staphylococcus aureus skin and soft tissue infections. Vaccine 2016;34:6402–7.

101. Chen L, He H, Wang M, et al. Surface coating of polytetrafluoroethylene with extracellular matrix and anti-CD34 antibodies facilitates endothelialization and inhibits platelet adhesion under sheer stress. Tissue Eng Regen Med 2017; 14:359–70.

102. Naito Y, Shinoka T, Duncan D, et al. Vascular tissue engineering: towards the next generation vascular grafts. Adv Drug Deliv Rev 2011;63:312–23.

103. Bratzler DW, Houck PM, Surgical Infection Prevention Guideline Writers Workgroup. Antimicrobial prophylaxis for surgery: an advisory statement from the National Surgical Infection Prevention Project. Am J Surg 2005;189:395–404.

104. Harbarth S, Samore MH, Lichtenberg D, et al. Prolonged antibiotic prophylaxis after cardiovascular surgery and its effect on surgical site infections and antimicrobial resistance. Circulation 2000;101:2916–21.

105. Alexander JW, Solomkin JS, Edwards MJ. Updated recommendations for control of surgical site infections. Ann Surg 2011;253:1082–93.

106. Anderson DJ, Podgorny K, Berrios-Torres SI, et al. Strategies to prevent surgical site infections in acute care hospitals: 2014 update. Infect Control Hosp Epidemiol 2014;35(Suppl 2):S66–88.
107. Weber WP, Mujagic E, Zwahlen M, et al. Timing of surgical antimicrobial prophylaxis: a phase 3 randomised controlled trial. Lancet Infect Dis 2017;17: 605–14.
108. Friberg Ö, Svedjeholm R, Söderquist B, et al. Local gentamicin reduces sternal wound infections after cardiac surgery: a randomized controlled trial. Ann Thorac Surg 2005;79:153–61.
109. Rutten H, Nijhuis P. Prevention of wound infection in elective colorectal surgery by local application of a gentamicin-containing collagen sponge. Eur J Surg Suppl 1997;(578):31–5.
110. Almeida CEPC, Reis L, Carvalho L, et al. Collagen implant with gentamicin sulphate reduces surgical site infection in vascular surgery: a prospective cohort study. Int J Surg 2014;12:1100–4.
111. Stewart AH, Eyers PS, Earnshaw JJ. Prevention of infection in peripheral arterial reconstruction: a systematic review and meta-analysis. J Vasc Surg 2007;46: 148–55.
112. Matatov T, Reddy KN, Doucet LD, et al. Experience with a new negative pressure incision management system in prevention of groin wound infection in vascular surgery patients. J Vasc Surg 2013;57:791–5.
113. Lee K, Murphy PB, Ingves MV, et al. Randomized clinical trial of negative pressure wound therapy for high-risk groin wounds in lower extremity revascularization. J Vasc Surg 2017;66(6):1814–9.

Cardiovascular Implantable Electronic Device Infections

Christopher J. Arnold, MD[a], Vivian H. Chu, MD, MHS[b],*

KEYWORDS

- Cardiovascular implantable electronic devices • Infection • Endocarditis
- Pacemaker • Implantable cardioverter defibrillator

KEY POINTS

- Cardiac device infection rates are increasing.
- *Staphylococcus* spp are the predominant causative organisms.
- Blood cultures, pocket tissue cultures, lead cultures, and echocardiography are key components of the diagnostic evaluation.
- Complete device extraction is a key component of management.
- Duration of antibiotic therapy and timing of device reimplantation vary depending on extent of infection.

INTRODUCTION

Cardiovascular disease is highly prevalent in the global population and thus there is an increasing population now living with cardiac implantable electronic devices (CIEDs). CIED infections (CDIs) are a serious potential complication, resulting in significant morbidity, mortality, and health care costs. Untreated, mortality approaches 66% and, even with appropriate therapy, the 1-year mortality remains as high as 18% to 20%.[1,2] The average length of hospital stay is approximately 2 weeks and recent data have shown mean hospitalization charges increasing to more than $170,000 over the past decade.[3] As such, understanding this complex infection, including its management and prevention, is of significant importance.

Disclosure Statement: Dr V.H. Chu reports grants from the National Institutes of Health: 1R34-AI122958-01, 4UL1-TR001117-04, 4R25-HD076475-04, 1R25-HL135304-01A1; consulting for Theravance; and authorship in UpToDate.

[a] Division of Infectious Diseases and International Health, University of Virginia Health System, PO Box 800545, Charlottesville, VA 22908-0545, USA; [b] Division of Infectious Diseases, Duke University Hospital, Duke Box 102359, Durham, NC 27710, USA
* Corresponding author.
E-mail address: vivian.chu@duke.edu

EPIDEMIOLOGY AND RISK FACTORS

With growing evidence to support the use of CIEDs to improve survival among patients with cardiac disease, the last 2 decades have seen a steady growth in implantations of these devices.[1] As of the second millennium, more than 3 million people worldwide were living with implanted cardiac electronic devices, including more than 180,000 implantable cardiac defibrillators (ICDs).[4] Since then, rates of placement have continued steady upward trends. More than 300,000 new CIEDs per year are placed in the United States alone, with more than 4 million people having had devices placed between the years 1993 and 2008.[2,5]

The increase in CIED implantations has been accompanied by a concomitant increase in CDIs. Rates of CDI are difficult to evaluate prospectively owing to the need for prolonged follow-up because infections can occur up to years following device implantation.[6,7] Duval and colleagues[6] reported as many as one-third of cardiac device–associated infective endocarditis (IE) cases occurred more than 3 years after the last device procedure. Thus, there is significant variation in the literature, with reported rates of CDI ranging from 0.13% to 19.9%.[4,8] In general, most recent studies report rates of 1% to 2%.[4,9–11] Rates vary depending on the type of infection (endocarditis vs pocket infection), devices reported (pacemakers [PMs] vs ICDs vs cardiac resynchronization devices), and duration of follow-up. CIED IE rates have generally been reported as between 1 and 2 per 1000 device years.[7,12–16] Many studies have found a higher rate of infection with more complex devices, such as ICDs or cardiac resynchronization therapy (CRT) devices, with rates of infection as much as 2 to 5 times higher than with PMs.[11,12,14,16] This may be because these devices are larger, thus requiring larger incisions, implantation pockets with more skin tension and larger potential dead space, and longer procedural times. Furthermore, these devices are often placed in patients with more comorbidities, which may affect risk for infection.[10,14]

Notably, the rates of CDI seem to be increasing out of proportion to that of device implantation.[11,17–20] One study reported a 96% increase in CIED implants over a 15-year period in the United States that was accompanied by a 210% increase in the CDI rate, from 1.5% to 2.4%.[10,20] Athan[21] reported a similar 200% increase between the years 2004 and 2008 using ICD coding in the US health care services. Toyoda and colleagues[15] found an increase in the rate of CIED IE from 1.3% to 4.1% between the years 1998 and 2013 in the states of California and New York. Another study reported an increase in incidence of CIED IE from 1.4 per 1000 implants in 1987 to 4.5 per 1000 implants in 2013. This resulted in an increase in the proportion of IE due to cardiac devices from 1.25% to 9.32% of all IE cases.[13] The precise reason for this disproportionate increase in the rate of CDI is not completely clear but it is likely multifactorial. With advances in medical technology and improvement in implantation techniques has come the opportunity to place devices in older patients, with many recent studies showing the average age of patients with CIED and CDIs as 70 years or older. These patients often have multiple comorbidities, many of which have been found to be risk factors for subsequent infection (see later discussion).[1,3,10,11,16] Additionally, the rates of implantation of more complex devices, including ICDs and CRTs has risen more steeply in recent years and, as previously suggested, these may have a higher rate of infection.[14]

Risk factors for CDI have been examined in numerous studies. A recent meta-analysis by Polyzos and colleagues[10] evaluated 60 different studies. In general, the risk factors are categorized as related to the patient, procedure, or device (**Box 1**). Most studies report a significant male predominance.[3,7,13,21] Comorbidities have

---

Box 1
Risk factors for cardiac implantable electronic devices

Patient

Diabetes mellitus

Chronic renal insufficiency

End-stage renal disease

Chronic obstructive pulmonary disease

History of previous device infection

Malignancy

Heart failure

Fever before procedure

Use of anticoagulation

Skin disorders

Procedure

Procedure duration

Hematoma

Need for reintervention or repeat device manipulation

Need for temporary pacing before implantation

Inexperienced operator

Lack of prophylactic periprocedural antibiotics

Device

Abdominal pocket

Epicardial leads

More than 1 lead

Dual-chamber system

CRT device

Data from Polyzos KA, Konstantelias AA, Falagas ME. Risk factors for cardiac implantable electronic device infection: a systematic review and meta-analysis. Europace 2015;17(5):767–77.

---

been shown to convey increased risk, including diabetes mellitus and chronic renal insufficiency.[3,7,10,14,21,22] Patients on dialysis not only have altered immunity but also require frequent vascular access procedures, which increase their risk of bacteremia.[11] The use of anticoagulation has been associated with higher risk of infection and likely relates to an increased risk of pocket hematoma, a procedure-related risk factor.[10]

Procedure-related risk factors include factors related to the procedure itself, as well as complications thereafter (see **Box 1**). Studies have suggested the protective effect of prophylactic and periprocedural antibiotics, and the subsequent increased risk of infection if they are not used.[4,10,21] As previously mentioned, postprocedural hematoma has been shown to be associated with increased risk of subsequent infection.[10,11,21,23] This may be related to delayed wound healing or dehiscence, an increased need for reintervention, and/or the fertile breeding ground for bacteria created by the hematoma. Indeed, perhaps among the strongest risk factors reported in the literature is the need for repeated intervention. Johansen and colleagues[7] found a nearly 3-fold increase in rate of infection following a device replacement compared with initial placement, with rate increasing from 1.82 per 1000 PM years to 5.32 per 1000 PM years. Multiple other studies have underscored a higher risk of infection with subsequent reentries into the pocket of the device.[4,9–11,14,16,21,23] This can include need for generator replacement, lead revision, hematoma evacuation, or other device revision.

Finally, device-associated risk factors tend to be associated with increased complexity of the devices. Higher numbers of leads, dual chamber systems, and abdominal pockets have all been associated with higher rates of CDI.[10,16,21,23] ICDs and CRTs seem to carry higher risks of CDI, including higher rates of CIED IE than PMs.[16]

MICROBIOLOGY

Gram-positive pathogens predominate in CDI, both in early-onset (<1 year from last device manipulation) and late-onset infection. Coagulase-negative staphylococci (CoNS) and Staphylococcus aureus remain the most common pathogens, accounting for 70% to 80% of infections in many series.[6,12,13,21,24–27] Several studies have suggested an increase in the incidence of methicillin resistance in the isolates causing CDI. For example, a recent study from the Cleveland Clinic showed a 15% incidence of methicillin-resistant Staphylococcus aureus (MRSA) between 2000 and 2011, up from 4% in a prior study reported at the Mayo Clinic.[25,28] In this study, 1 in every 3 CDIs was due to a methicillin-resistant staphylococcal organism, which is consistent with other series.[24,27] Thus, empiric antimicrobial therapy for CDI should include coverage for methicillin-resistant gram-positive pathogens while awaiting a microbiological diagnosis.

CoNS are statistically the most common pathogens in CDI; therefore, the isolation of CoNS from the blood or device pocket should be taken seriously and carefully evaluated rather than dismissed as contaminants. These biofilm producers are frequently associated with foreign body infection and are adept at evading the immune system. Biofilm exopolymer production by CoNS may protect from antibody recognition and promote resistance to phagocytosis.[29] Although most studies show them to be the most common causative organisms irrespective of timing of onset of infection, CoNS have a strong association with late-onset generator pocket infections. CoNS are less often associated with endovascular infection than is Staphylococcus aureus.[24,25]

Staphylococcus aureus is the most common pathogen associated with endovascular infection involving CIEDs, and is more likely than CoNS to present with systemic signs and symptoms of infection.[29] Several studies have underscored the strong association of Staphylococcus aureus bacteremia (SAB) with underlying CDI.[28,30] Chamis and colleagues[30] showed a 45.4% incidence of confirmed CDI in all subjects with SAB and a CIED present. Early SAB (<1 year after last device manipulation) was more highly associated with confirmed CDI than was late SAB (75% vs 28.5%). However, the incidence of CDI in late SAB increased to 71.5% when including cases of possible CDI. This study found that in early SAB, the CIED was often the primary source of bacteremia as opposed to late SAB in which device involvement was often from hematogenous seeding from a distant site. Importantly, up to 60% of those with confirmed CDI had no local signs or symptoms to suggest pocket infection; with up to 50% of these still having positive pocket cultures. Taken together, the results suggest that clinicians must have a high index of suspicion for CDI in the presence of SAB, even with negative echocardiographic findings and no local signs or symptoms at the generator pocket. On this basis, the investigators of the aforementioned study proposed device removal for patients with SAB, irrespective of negative echocardiogram or physical examination findings in patients without an alternative identifiable source of SAB or in those with relapsing bacteremia.

Gram-negative pathogens are infrequent causes of CDI, accounting for 6% to 9% of infections in most series.[8,24–27] A 7-year retrospective study done at the Mayo Clinic showed that only 6% of subjects with gram-negative bacteremia (GNB) had definite (n = 2) or possible (n = 1) CDI. The 2 subjects found to have definite CDI had obvious signs of pocket infection. In those with GNB who retained their CIEDs, only 2 had relapse of bacteremia and in both there was an obvious alternative source.[8] A more recent study at Duke University Hospital aimed to stratify risk among various bacterial species.[31] This study showed higher rates of CDI in subjects bacteremic with *Pseudomonas aeruginosa* (53.8%) and *Serratia marcescens* (46.7%), with rates approaching that of *Staphylococcus aureus* (54.6%). All other gram-negative pathogens showed a low incidence consistent with prior studies (7.6%). It should be noted that a high percentage of the subjects with *Pseudomonas* and *Serratia* infections had left-ventricular assist devices (LVADs) in situ, which is outside of the scope of devices included in this review. In light of these studies, it would be reasonable for clinicians to have a low index of suspicion for CDI in patients with GNB and no local signs of pocket infection. More careful attention should be paid to those with *Pseudomonas* or *Serratia* bacteremia without an obvious alternative source, particularly if they have an LVAD in situ.

A variety of other pathogens can cause CDI. Aside from CoNS, other common skin flora, such as *Propionibacterium acnes* and *Corynebacterium* spp, have been shown to play a significant role.[24] As such, the isolation of these microorganisms should be carefully evaluated before considering them as contaminants. Fungal CDI is rare but has been seen with a variety of both yeasts and molds. Additionally, there are reports of infections with various atypical mycobacterial species. A summary of these uncommon causes can be found in prior reviews.[32]

CLINICAL MANIFESTATIONS

CDI are generally categorized as being either superficial (pocket) or deep (lead and/or valvular). Generator pocket infections are the most common and often present with local signs of inflammation at the generator pocket site, which can include pain, swelling, erythema, warmth, and dehiscence with or without drainage. Although pocket infections can be associated with bacteremia and systemic symptoms, more commonly they present without bacteremia or systemic symptoms.[26,33,34] Some may present only with erosion of the generator through the skin. In this circumstance, even in the absence of other concerning signs or symptoms, the device is considered infected and should be managed accordingly.[34] Traditionally, pocket infections have been said to occur soon after device implantation or manipulation, likely due to contamination of the pocket in or around the time of the procedure. However, some recent studies have shown almost half of pocket infections to occur more than 1 year after the last device manipulation.[5,35] In a recent study comparing early to late pocket infections, early infections were found to be more likely to present with inflammatory changes at the pocket site versus late infections that were more likely to present as device erosion. There was no difference in the incidence of lead vegetations between the 2 groups, although valvular vegetations were more commonly seen in the setting of late pocket infection.[35]

Deep infection refers to involvement of either the transvenous portion of the lead and the continuous endocardium or valve, or the epicardial electrode and the contiguous epicardium. These infections are more likely to be associated with bacteremia and systemic symptoms. Fevers and chills are present more often than not, occurring in at least 80% of patients.[21] The clinical presentation is often similar to valvular endocarditis and, similar to subacute bacterial endocarditis, the diagnosis is often delayed due to nonspecific signs and symptoms.[36] Recurrent pulmonary infections and/or pulmonary radiographic abnormalities (pneumonia, lung abscess, embolism) are not uncommon, occurring in 20% to 45% of patients.[6,36–40] These infections can be seen in conjunction with concomitant pocket infection and thus the presence of pocket infection with systemic symptoms or positive blood cultures should prompt evaluation for deeper extension of infection.

DIAGNOSIS AND DIAGNOSTIC TESTING

Diagnosis is fairly straightforward in those patients presenting with overt signs of inflammation, dehiscence, or erosion at the generator pocket site. One caveat is with patients presenting within the first 30 days postimplantation with erythema of the pocket, which can sometimes be reflective of early postimplantation inflammation or superficial incisional infection as opposed to true device infection. In this circumstance, if there is no purulent exudate, dehiscence, fluctuance, or systemic signs of infection, then these patients may be managed with very close follow-up and sometimes a short course of oral antibiotic therapy, with the knowledge that symptoms should resolve within 2 weeks. In all other cases, however, a presumptive clinical diagnosis is made and can be confirmed via culture of tissue and purulent fluid from the pocket. Tissue cultures obtained during surgical exploration are more sensitive than swab cultures.[33] Percutaneous aspiration of the pocket should not be performed due to lower diagnostic yield and the theoretic risk of introduction of bacteria into the pocket that could cause subsequent infection.[33] Additionally, at least 2 sets (and preferably 3 sets if there is a high suspicion for CIED IE) of blood cultures should be obtained before the initiation of antimicrobial therapy. Previous studies have shown the yield of blood cultures in the diagnosis of all CDIs to be between 33% to 40%, and this climbs to more than 80% in cases of CIED IE.[21,20,32,37,38,11] Additionally, cultures of the lead tips should be sent following device extraction. Microbiologic yield from these cultures have been reported to be as high as 50% to 90%.[21,40] Some recent studies have suggested that sonification of the leads and generator devices following removal may increase the microbiologic yield.[44–47] Importantly, when leads have been extracted through the pocket, a positive lead tip culture may reflect contamination by the pocket and not true lead-associated endocarditis. Thus, these cultures need to be interpreted carefully. In patients with negative blood cultures and no concerning echocardiographic findings, positive lead tip cultures should not be erroneously interpreted because this can result in unduly long courses of antibiotic therapy and associated toxicities.[33,38]

The presence of systemic symptoms or positive blood cultures should prompt further evaluation for deeper infection with echocardiography.[33] Numerous studies have shown that transesophageal echocardiography (TEE) is more sensitive than is transthoracic echocardiography (TTE) for detection of vegetations.[1,13,21,27,28,30,36,48–50] Thus a negative TTE should be followed up with a TEE to assess for lead and/or valvular vegetations. Notably, the sensitivity of TEE is not 100%; thus a negative TEE cannot definitively rule out CIED IE. Several studies have suggested that if generator pocket abnormalities and pulmonary embolism are added to the Modified Duke Criteria, there is a significant increase in the diagnostic value of these criteria for CIED IE.[36,40]

Recent studies have shown high sensitivity and specificity for determination of CDI using fluorine-18 fluorodeoxyglucose PET–computed tomography (^{18}F-FDG PET-CT) imaging.[51–56] A meta-analysis that included 340 subjects showed a pooled sensitivity and specificity of 87% and 94%, respectively. The sensitivity and specificity are noted to be higher for determining pocket infection (93% and 98%, respectively) than for CIED IE (65% and 88%, respectively).[56] Although the evidence to date is insufficient for ^{18}F-FDG PET-CT to have been included in the guidelines, the available data suggest that it may be a helpful adjunctive test. It may be particularly useful in cases in which there is question regarding early postimplantation inflammation versus pocket infection, as well as in cases in which suspicion is high for deeper infection but other modalities such as echocardiography have been negative.[34]

MANAGEMENT

Superficial infections of the skin that do not involve the pocket can be managed with oral antibiotics alone without device removal. In these cases, patients can be treated with 7 to 10 days of an oral antibiotic regimen with antistaphylococcal activity, coupled with close observation to ensure no signs or symptoms of deeper extension develop.[26,32,33,40,42] For all confirmed CDIs, complete device extraction is recommended as first-line therapy.[33] Multiple studies have shown higher clinical failure and relapse rates when treatment with device retention is attempted.[32–34,42,57–59] In a retrospective study of 416 subjects with CDIs, there was a 7-fold increase in 30-day mortality in those treated with antimicrobial therapy alone without device removal. In this same study, early device removal coupled with antimicrobial therapy was associated with a 3-fold decrease in 1-year mortality.[60] A more recent retrospective study looked at chronic suppressive antibiotic therapy in subjects who did not undergo device removal. The median overall survival in these subjects was 1.43 years, with 18% of subjects developing relapse in 1 year.[61] This study suggests this as a possible alternative for patients who cannot undergo device removal. The current guidelines recommend this approach only in cases in which device removal is deemed not possible.[33]

When considering device removal, these should be performed at centers that have immediate availability of cardiothoracic surgery to intervene should complications arise.[33,34] Percutaneous device removal is favored to surgical removal. There is a debate in the literature in regard to the need for surgical removal in patients with larger vegetations (>2 cm) to minimize risk of resultant pulmonary embolism. Some investigators have more recently suggested that even devices with larger vegetations can safely be removed percutaneously.[26] The most recent guidelines suggest that each case should be individualized with respect to this given the paucity of data.[33]

Antibiotic therapy is adjunctive to device removal. Because there are no randomized clinical trial data to inform optimal duration of therapy, there is variation in practice observed. This was illustrated by a recent study in which infectious disease specialists were surveyed in regard to their practice.[62] Although some specialists' practices mirrored the guidelines, others showed significant variation in duration of antimicrobial therapy recommended. There are several published algorithms regarding duration of therapy (**Fig. 1**).[26,33,34] The current guidelines recommend 10 to 14 days of antimicrobial therapy for pocket infections without concomitant bacteremia. The recommended duration for those with bacteremia is a minimum of 14 days, which should be extended to at least 4 weeks if blood cultures remain positive after device removal. If there is bacteremia with concomitant evidence of vegetations on echocardiography, then therapy should be approached as in IE with 4 to 6 weeks of antimicrobial therapy.[33]

Careful reassessment of the need for the cardiac device should be undertaken before considering reimplantation. In a study, 33% of subjects were found to have no further need for ongoing cardiac device on reevaluation.[26] The optimal timing of device replacement after removal is not known. **Fig. 2** depicts a proposed algorithm for

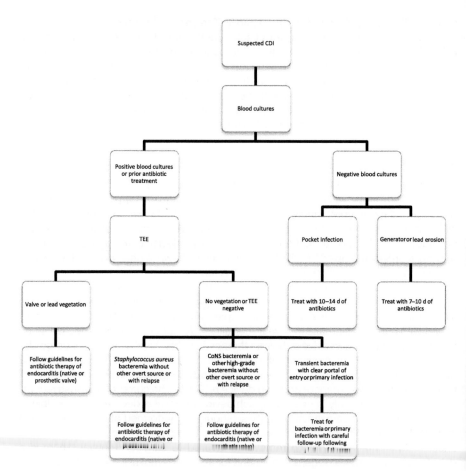

Fig. 1. Approach to antibiotic management of adults with CDI. (*Adapted from* Sohail MR, Uslan DZ, Khan AH, et al. Management and outcome of permanent pacemaker and implantable cardioverter-defibrillator infections. J Am Coll Cardiol 2007;49:1851; with permission.)

device reimplantation.[26,33] One center described simultaneous contralateral replacement of infected CIEDs in 68 subjects with good success[63]; however, there are insufficient corroborating studies to recommend this approach presently. The current guidelines recommend ensuring negative blood cultures for at least 72 hours before replacement. This is extended to 14 days if there are valvular vegetations seen on echocardiography.[33] It is recommended that the device be replaced on the contralateral side from the current infection.[33]

PREVENTION

Periprocedural antimicrobial prophylaxis has been shown in multiple studies to reduce risk of subsequent infection.[4,26,32,33,64,65] One large randomized, double-blind, placebo-controlled trial of preprocedural cefazolin was halted early when an interim analysis showed a substantial benefit (0.63% vs 3.28% infection rate).[65] The antibiotic chosen should have staphylococcal activity, and most investigators advocate for the continued use of first-generation cephalosporins. Vancomycin provides an

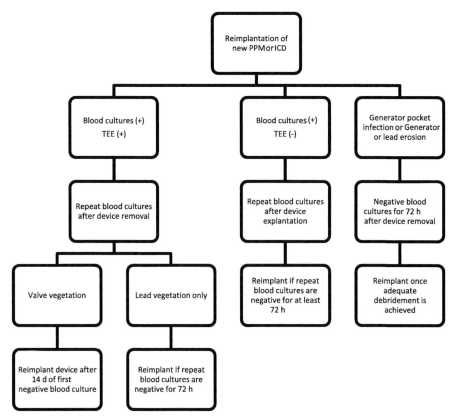

Fig. 2. Approach to device reimplantation in CDI. −, negative; +, positive; PPM, permanent PM. (*From* Sohail MR, Uslan DZ, Khan AH, et al. Management and outcome of permanent pacemaker and implantable cardioverter-defibrillator infections. J Am Coll Cardiol 2007;49:1851; with permission.)

alternative for patients with beta-lactam allergies. Cefazolin should be administered within 1 hour before the procedure as opposed to vancomycin that, if used, should be given within 2 hours prior.[33] Postprocedural antibiotics are not recommended given the lack of evidence to show further benefit and the risks of ongoing antibiotic therapy.

Antibiotic prophylaxis before invasive procedures that are not directly related to CIED manipulation (ie, dental, gastrointestinal, genitourinary, dermatologic) is not recommended based on limited evidence to show benefit and potential associated risks. A review of more than 140 articles published between 1950 and 2007 showed no reports of hematogenous infection from among the aforementioned procedures.[33] Furthermore, the predominant pathogens in CDIs are staphylococci, which would not be the expected pathogen associated with translocation during dental, gastrointestinal, or genitourinary procedures.

More recently, there has been interest in antimicrobial eluting bacterial envelopes to help prevent infection. The TYRX (Medtronic, Monmouth Junction, NJ) antibacterial envelope is a monofilament polypropylene mesh that holds the CIED in place and emits rifampin and minocycline slowly over time. Noncontrolled studies showed infection rate reduction with its use.[66–68] More recently, 2 large multicenter prospective cohort studies were conducted to evaluate its efficacy. These studies showed a very low infection rate of 0.4%, which was significantly lower than the 12-month benchmark rate of 2.2%. A reduction was seen in all subgroups including in those with CRT and ICD devices.[69]

Finally, advances in device technology continue with the advent of epicardial lead systems, subcutaneous ICD (S-ICD), and leadless PM systems. With these advances there are the hopes of potential infection reduction, particularly for those patients at risk for recurrent bacteremia, such as hemodialysis (HD) patients. One small study evaluated HD subjects who had experienced CDI with transvenous-lead ICD (T-ICD) systems, which were then subsequently replaced with an epicardial system. Although the 6 subjects experienced, on average, 1.5 episodes of dialysis catheter-related bacteremia over more than 1 year of follow-up, none developed infection of the epicardial system.[70] Although, this suggests epicardial systems may provide an avenue of reduced risk for HD patients, a recent systematic review identified epicardial leads as a risk factor for CDI.[10] More recently, S-ICD systems, in which the entire device and leads are entirely extravascular, have been developed.[71–73] Unfortunately, the data regarding potential for infection reduction with this approach has been conflicting. Infection rates have ranged from 5% to 10%, with the larger studies reporting rates most consistently around 5%.[73] The rate of pocket infection seems to be higher with the S-ICD systems, possibly related to the 3 incisions required for placement.[73] Although further advances in this area are expected, at this time, there is insufficient evidence to support S-ICD as a means to reduce infection rate.

An entirely intracardiac leadless PM system has also been developed. This system is nonsurgically implanted into the right ventricle with use of a catheter through the femoral vein.[74] Although this leadless system has the potential to reduce infection risk, substantive data regarding rates of infection are currently not available.

SUMMARY

Infections associated with CIEDs are increasing and are associated with significant morbidity and mortality. These infections are predominantly caused by gram-positive organisms, particularly staphylococci. *Staphylococcus aureus* bacteremia in the setting of a cardiac device often indicates CDI and should raise a high index of suspicion for infection. CDI can present as pocket infection with or without systemic symptoms, or as deeper infection involving the device leads and/or cardiac valves. Device erosion is, by default, considered infection and managed accordingly. Physical examination of the pocket site, blood cultures, pocket tissue cultures, lead tip cultures, and echocardiography are all important components of diagnosis, although ^{18}F-FDG PET-CT may play in a role in some cases in which the initial work-up is inconclusive. Complete device extraction is an important part of the management of CDI, along with adjunctive antibiotic therapy. The duration of antibiotic therapy can range from 7 days to 6 weeks, depending on extent of infection. Preoperative antibiotics are a mainstay strategy for reducing infection rates. Technological advances, such as antibacterial envelopes and novel cardiac devices, provide potential avenues for future risk reduction.

REFERENCES

1. Tarakji KG, Wazni OM, Harb S, et al. Risk factors for 1-year mortality among patients with cardiac implantable electronic device infection undergoing transvenous lead extraction: the impact of the infection type and the presence of vegetation on survival. Europace 2014;16(10):1490–5.

2. Hussein A, Tarakji K, Martin D, et al. Cardiac implantable electronic device infections: added complexity and suboptimal outcomes with previously abandoned leads. JACC Clin Electrophysiol 2017;3(1):1–9.
3. Sridhar AR, Lavu M, Yarlagadda V, et al. Cardiac implantable electronic device-related infection and extraction trends in the U.S. Pacing Clin Electrophysiol 2017;40(3):286–93.
4. Klug D, Balde M, Pavin D, et al. Risk factors related to infections of implanted pacemakers and cardioverter-defibrillators: results of a large prospective study. Circulation 2007;116(12):1349–55.
5. Tarakji KG, Wilkoff BL. Cardiac implantable electronic device infections: facts, current practice, and the unanswered questions. Curr Infect Dis Rep 2014; 16(9):425.
6. Duval X, Selton-Suty C, Alla F, et al. Endocarditis in patients with a permanent pacemaker: a 1-year epidemiological survey on infective endocarditis due to valvular and/or pacemaker infection. Clin Infect Dis 2004;39(1):68–74.
7. Johansen JB, Jorgensen OD, Moller M, et al. Infection after pacemaker implantation: infection rates and risk factors associated with infection in a population-based cohort study of 46299 consecutive patients. Eur Heart J 2011;32(8):991–8.
8. Uslan DZ, Sohail MR, Friedman PA, et al. Frequency of permanent pacemaker or implantable cardioverter-defibrillator infection in patients with gram-negative bacteremia. Clin Infect Dis 2006;43(6):731–6.
9. Rahman R, Saba S, Bazaz R, et al. Infection and readmission rate of cardiac implantable electronic device insertions: an observational single center study. Am J Infect Control 2016;44(3):278–82.
10. Polyzos KA, Konstantelias AA, Falagas ME. Risk factors for cardiac implantable electronic device infection: a systematic review and meta-analysis. Europace 2015;17(5):767–77.
11. Prutkin JM, Reynolds MR, Bao H, et al. Rates of and factors associated with infection in 200 909 Medicare implantable cardioverter-defibrillator implants: results from the National Cardiovascular Data Registry. Circulation 2014;130(13): 1037–43.
12. Uslan DZ, Sohail MR, St Sauver JL, et al. Permanent pacemaker and implantable cardioverter defibrillator infection: a population-based study. Arch Intern Med 2007;167(7):669–75.
13. Carrasco F, Anguita M, Ruiz M, et al. Clinical features and changes in epidemiology of infective endocarditis on pacemaker devices over a 27-year period (1987-2013). Europace 2016;18(6):836–41.
14. Ann HW, Ahn JY, Jeon YD, et al. Incidence of and risk factors for infectious complications in patients with cardiac device implantation. Int J Infect Dis 2015;36: 9–14.
15. Toyoda N, Chikwe J, Itagaki S, et al. Trends in infective endocarditis in California and New York State, 1998-2013. JAMA 2017;317(16):1652–60.
16. Ozcan C, Raunso J, Lamberts M, et al. Infective endocarditis and risk of death after cardiac implantable electronic device implantation: a nationwide cohort study. Europace 2017;19(6):1007–14.
17. Voigt A, Shalaby A, Saba S. Rising rates of cardiac rhythm management device infections in the United States: 1996 through 2003. J Am Coll Cardiol 2006;48(3): 590–1.
18. Voigt A, Shalaby A, Saba S. Continued rise in rates of cardiovascular implantable electronic device infections in the United States: temporal trends and causative insights. Pacing Clin Electrophysiol 2010;33(4):414–9.

19. Cabell CH, Heidenreich PA, Chu VH, et al. Increasing rates of cardiac device infections among Medicare beneficiaries: 1990-1999. Am Heart J 2004;147(4): 582–6.

20. Greenspon AJ, Patel JD, Lau E, et al. 16-year trends in the infection burden for pacemakers and implantable cardioverter-defibrillators in the United States 1993 to 2008. J Am Coll Cardiol 2011;58(10):1001–6.

21. Athan E. The characteristics and outcome of infective endocarditis involving implantable cardiac devices. Curr Infect Dis Rep 2014;16(12):446.

22. Habib A, Le KY, Baddour LM, et al. Predictors of mortality in patients with cardiovascular implantable electronic device infections. Am J Cardiol 2013;111(6): 874–9.

23. Raad D, Irani J, Akl EG, et al. Implantable electrophysiologic cardiac device infections: a risk factor analysis. Eur J Clin Microbiol Infect Dis 2012;31(11): 3015–21.

24. Bongiorni MG, Tascini C, Tagliaferri E, et al. Microbiology of cardiac implantable electronic device infections. Europace 2012;14(9):1334–9.

25. Hussein A, Baghdy Y, Wazni O, et al. Microbiology of cardiac implantable electronic device infections. JACC Clin Electrophysiol 2016;2(4):498–505.

26. Sohail MR, Uslan DZ, Khan AH, et al. Management and outcome of permanent pacemaker and implantable cardioverter-defibrillator infections. J Am Coll Cardiol 2007;49(18):1851–9.

27. Tarakji KG, Chan EJ, Cantillon DJ, et al. Cardiac implantable electronic device infections: presentation, management, and patient outcomes. Heart Rhythm 2010; 7(8):1043–7.

28. Uslan DZ, Dowsley TF, Sohail MR, et al. Cardiovascular implantable electronic device infection in patients with *Staphylococcus aureus* bacteremia. Pacing Clin Electrophysiol 2010;33(4):407–13.

29. Le KY, Sohail MR, Friedman PA, et al. Clinical features and outcomes of cardiovascular implantable electronic device infections due to staphylococcal species. Am J Cardiol 2012;110(8):1143–9.

30. Chamis AL, Peterson GE, Cabell CH, et al. *Staphylococcus aureus* bacteremia in patients with permanent pacemakers or implantable cardioverter-defibrillators. Circulation 2001;104(9):1029–33.

31. Maskarinec SA, Thaden JT, Cyr DD, et al. The risk of cardiac device-related infection in bacteremic patients is species specific: results of a 12-year prospective cohort. Open Forum Infect Dis 2017;4(3):ofx132.

32. Gandhi T, Crawford T, Riddell J 4th. Cardiovascular implantable electronic device associated infections. Infect Dis Clin North Am 2012;26(1):57–76.

33. Baddour LM, Epstein AE, Erickson CC, et al. Update on cardiovascular implantable electronic device infections and their management: a scientific statement from the American Heart Association. Circulation 2010;121(3):458–77.

34. Sandoe JA, Barlow G, Chambers JB, et al. Guidelines for the diagnosis, prevention and management of implantable cardiac electronic device infection. Report of a joint Working Party project on behalf of the British Society for Antimicrobial Chemotherapy (BSAC, host organization), British Heart Rhythm Society (BHRS), British Cardiovascular Society (BCS), British Heart Valve Society (BHVS) and British Society for Echocardiography (BSE). J Antimicrob Chemother 2015;70(2):325–59.

35. Welch M, Uslan DZ, Greenspon AJ, et al. Variability in clinical features of early versus late cardiovascular implantable electronic device pocket infections. Pacing Clin Electrophysiol 2014;37(8):955–62.

36. Polewczyk A, Janion M, Podlaski R, et al. Clinical manifestations of lead-dependent infective endocarditis: analysis of 414 cases. Eur J Clin Microbiol Infect Dis 2014;33(9):1601–8.
37. Massoure PL, Reuter S, Lafitte S, et al. Pacemaker endocarditis: clinical features and management of 60 consecutive cases. Pacing Clin Electrophysiol 2007; 30(1):12–9.
38. Sohail MR, Uslan DZ, Khan AH, et al. Infective endocarditis complicating permanent pacemaker and implantable cardioverter-defibrillator infection. Mayo Clin Proc 2008;83(1):46–53.
39. Cacoub P, Leprince P, Nataf P, et al. Pacemaker infective endocarditis. Am J Cardiol 1998;82(4):480–4.
40. Klug D, Lacroix D, Savoye C, et al. Systemic infection related to endocarditis on pacemaker leads: clinical presentation and management. Circulation 1997;95(8): 2098–107.
41. Cengiz M, Okutucu S, Ascioglu S, et al. Permanent pacemaker and implantable cardioverter defibrillator infections: seven years of diagnostic and therapeutic experience of a single center. Clin Cardiol 2010;33(7):406–11.
42. Chua JD, Wilkoff BL, Lee I, et al. Diagnosis and management of infections involving implantable electrophysiologic cardiac devices. Ann Intern Med 2000; 133(8):604–8.
43. Grammes JA, Schulze CM, Al-Bataineh M, et al. Percutaneous pacemaker and implantable cardioverter-defibrillator lead extraction in 100 patients with intracardiac vegetations defined by transesophageal echocardiogram. J Am Coll Cardiol 2010;55(9):886–94.
44. Rohacek M, Erne P, Kobza R, et al. Infection of cardiovascular implantable electronic devices: detection with sonication, swab cultures, and blood cultures. Pacing Clin Electrophysiol 2015;38(2):247–53.
45. Rohacek M, Weisser M, Kobza R, et al. Bacterial colonization and infection of electrophysiological cardiac devices detected with sonication and swab culture. Circulation 2010;121(15):1691–7.
46. Inacio RC, Klautau GB, Murca MA, et al. Microbial diagnosis of infection and colonization of cardiac implantable electronic devices by use of sonication. Int J Infect Dis 2015;38:54–9.
47. Oliva A, Nguyen BL, Mascellino MT, et al. Sonication of explanted cardiac implants improves microbial detection in cardiac device infections. J Clin Microbiol 2013;51(2):496–502.
48. van Hoff R, Friedman H. Implantable cardioverter-defibrillator and pacemaker infections. Hosp Med Clin 2015;4(2):150–62.
49. Sohail MR, Palraj BR, Khalid S, et al. Predicting risk of endovascular device infection in patients with Staphylococcus aureus bacteremia (PREDICT-SAB). Circ Arrhythm Electrophysiol 2015;8(1):137–44.
50. Golzio PG, Fanelli AL, Vinci M, et al. Lead vegetations in patients with local and systemic cardiac device infections: prevalence, risk factors, and therapeutic effects. Europace 2013;15(1):89–100.
51. Pizzi MN, Dos-Subira L, Roque A, et al. 18F-FDG-PET/CT angiography in the diagnosis of infective endocarditis and cardiac device infection in adult patients with congenital heart disease and prosthetic material. Int J Cardiol 2017;248: 396–402.
52. Tlili G, Amraoui S, Mesguich C, et al. High performances of (18)F-fluorodeoxyglucose PET-CT in cardiac implantable device infections: a study of 40 patients. J Nucl Cardiol 2015;22(4):787–98.

53. Ahmed FZ, James J, Cunnington C, et al. Early diagnosis of cardiac implantable electronic device generator pocket infection using (1)(8)F-FDG-PET/CT. Eur Heart J Cardiovasc Imaging 2015;16(5):521–30.
54. Graziosi M, Nanni C, Lorenzini M, et al. Role of (1)(8)F-FDG PET/CT in the diagnosis of infective endocarditis in patients with an implanted cardiac device: a prospective study. Eur J Nucl Med Mol Imaging 2014;41(8):1617–23.
55. Sarrazin JF, Philippon F, Tessier M, et al. Usefulness of fluorine-18 positron emission tomography/computed tomography for identification of cardiovascular implantable electronic device infections. J Am Coll Cardiol 2012;59(18):1616–25.
56. Juneau D, Golfam M, Hazra S, et al. Positron emission tomography and single-photon emission computed tomography imaging in the diagnosis of cardiac implantable electronic device infection: a systematic review and meta-analysis. Circ Cardiovasc Imaging 2017;10(4) [pii:e005772].
57. Margey R, McCann H, Blake G, et al. Contemporary management of and outcomes from cardiac device related infections. Europace 2010;12(1):64–70.
58. van Herick A, Schuetz CA, Alperin P, et al. The impact of initial statin treatment decisions on cardiovascular outcomes in clinical care settings: estimates using the Archimedes Model. Clinicoecon Outcomes Res 2012;4:337–47.
59. Camus C, Leport C, Raffi F, et al. Sustained bacteremia in 26 patients with a permanent endocardial pacemaker: assessment of wire removal. Clin Infect Dis 1993;17(1):46–55.
60. Le KY, Sohail MR, Friedman PA, et al. Impact of timing of device removal on mortality in patients with cardiovascular implantable electronic device infections. Heart Rhythm 2011;8(11):1678–85.
61. Tan EM, DeSimone DC, Sohail MR, et al. Outcomes in patients with cardiovascular implantable electronic device infection managed with chronic antibiotic suppression. Clin Infect Dis 2017;64(11):1516–21.
62. Liang SY, Beekmann SE, Polgreen PM, et al. Current management of cardiac implantable electronic device infections by infectious disease specialists. Clin Infect Dis 2016;63(8):1072–9.
63. Nandyala R, Parsonnet V. One stage side-to-side replacement of infected pulse generators and leads. Pacing Clin Electrophysiol 2006;29(4):393–6.
64. Da Costa A, Kirkorian G, Cucherat M, et al. Antibiotic prophylaxis for permanent pacemaker implantation: a meta-analysis. Circulation 1998;97(18):1796–801.
65. de Oliveira JC, Martinelli M, Nishioka SA, et al. Efficacy of antibiotic prophylaxis before the implantation of pacemakers and cardioverter-defibrillators: results of a large, prospective, randomized, double-blinded, placebo-controlled trial. Circ Arrhythm Electrophysiol 2009;2(1):29–34.
66. Kolek MJ, Patel NJ, Clair WK, et al. Efficacy of a bio-absorbable antibacterial envelope to prevent cardiac implantable electronic device infections in high-risk subjects. J Cardiovasc Electrophysiol 2015;26(10):1111–6.
67. Bloom HL, Constantin L, Dan D, et al. Implantation success and infection in cardiovascular implantable electronic device procedures utilizing an antibacterial envelope. Pacing Clin Electrophysiol 2011;34(2):133–42.
68. Mittal S, Shaw RE, Michel K, et al. Cardiac implantable electronic device infections: incidence, risk factors, and the effect of the AigisRx antibacterial envelope. Heart Rhythm 2014;11(4):595–601.
69. Henrikson CA, Sohail MR, Acosta H, et al. Antibacterial envelope is associated with low infection rates after implantable cardioverter-defibrillator and cardiac resynchronization therapy device replacement. JACC Clin Electrophysiol 2017; 3(10):1158–67.

70. Asif A, Carrillo R, Garisto JD, et al. Epicardial cardiac rhythm devices for dialysis patients: minimizing the risk of infection and preserving central veins. Semin Dial 2012;25(1):88–94.
71. Olde Nordkamp LR, Dabiri Abkenari L, Boersma LV, et al. The entirely subcutaneous implantable cardioverter-defibrillator: initial clinical experience in a large Dutch cohort. J Am Coll Cardiol 2012;60(19):1933–9.
72. Weiss R, Knight BP, Gold MR, et al. Safety and efficacy of a totally subcutaneous implantable-cardioverter defibrillator. Circulation 2013;128(9):944–53.
73. Aziz S, Leon AR, El-Chami MF. The subcutaneous defibrillator: a review of the literature. J Am Coll Cardiol 2014;63(15):1473–9.
74. Reddy VY, Exner DV, Cantillon DJ, et al. Percutaneous implantation of an entirely intracardiac leadless pacemaker. N Engl J Med 2015;373(12):1125–35.

Ventricular Assist Device–Associated Infection

Tee K. Teoh, MD, Margaret M. Hannan, MD*

KEYWORDS

- VAD-related infections • VAD-specific infections • Non-VAD infections • Driveline
- Implantable cardiac device

KEY POINTS

- Despite the many advances in ventricular assist devices (VADs), infection still remains a major cause of morbidity and mortality.
- The International Society for Heart and Lung Transplant defined infections related to VAD permits analysis of the source and pathophysiology of left ventricular assist device (LVAD) infections in addition to guiding diagnosis and management of LVAD infections. Infections related to VADs are separated into 3 categories: VAD-specific infections, VAD-related infections, and non-VAD-related infections.
- The management of VAD-specific and VAD-related infections is highly individualized, and the input of an infection specialist who is familiar with such devices should be obtained in most cases. Early surgical opinion should be considered for surgical management.
- Prevention of infections related to VAD is important. Emphasis should be given for a comprehensive infection prevention and control program, intraoperative and perioperative measures, and drive-line care.

INTRODUCTION

The prevalence of heart failure is increasing worldwide due to an aging population and advances in therapeutic innovations for heart failure treatment resulting in increased survival. Heart failure remains a major contributor to morbidity and mortality worldwide. It is estimated that the total number of patients in the United States with heart failure is 5.1 million.[1] Cardiac transplantation is a potential life-saving treatment for patients with end-stage disease but relies on a very limited number of suitable donors.

Ventricular assist devices (VADs) are mechanical pumps that supplement or replace the function of damaged ventricles to maintain appropriate blood flow in patients with end-stage heart failure (**Fig. 1**). VADs can be right ventricular devices, left ventricular devices, and if both are implanted, biventricular assist devices, or total artificial hearts.

Department of Clinical Microbiology, Mater Misericordiae University Hospital, University College Dublin, Eccles Street, Dublin 7, Dublin, Ireland
* Corresponding author.
E-mail address: mhannan@mater.ie

Infect Dis Clin N Am 32 (2018) 827–841
https://doi.org/10.1016/j.idc.2018.07.001
id.theclinics.com

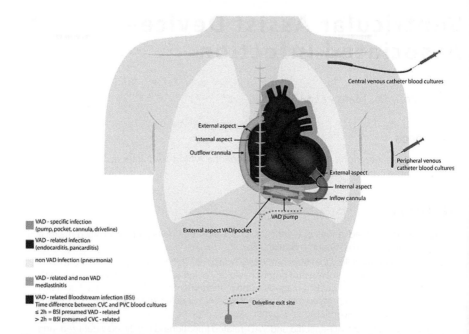

Fig. 1. VAD-specific, VAD-related, and non-VAD infection. CVC, central venous catheter; PVC, peripheral vascular catheter. (*From* Hannan M, Husain S, Mattner F, et al. Working formulation for the standardization of definitions of infections in patients using ventricular assist devices. J Heart Lung Transplant 2011;30(4):378; with permission.)

The most common is the left ventricular assist device (LVAD), and for this article, VAD is discussed as LVAD.[2,3] Largely, the principle of diagnosis, management, and treatment of infection in all VADs is similar. Although the use of LVADs was initially used as a bridge to transplant (BTT), there has been increasing expansion of the use to LVADs as a bridge to decision and as a permanent implant, a strategy known as destination therapy (DT).[2–5]

LVAD has been shown to be superior to maximal medical therapy in selected patient groups.[6] Successful LVAD conditioning has been shown to reduce admissions and hospitalization in end-stage heart failure patients.[7] However, LVADs are still associated with high complications rates.[2,3,8,9]

LEFT VENTRICULAR ASSIST DEVICES OVERVIEW/EPIDEMIOLOGY

Despite the advancement in therapy for heart failure, both medically and with mechanical circulatory support, cardiac transplant remains the definitive therapy for end-stage heart failure. Cardiac transplants, however, are limited by the availability of donor organs.

The LVAD was first conceived as an implantable mechanical support device for circulatory support in patients who have end-stage heart failure. The field of LVADs is a rapidly evolving area of medicine. Patients who undergo insertion of LVADs usually have worsening New York Heart Association (NYHA) class IIIb or class IV heart failure, typically despite inotropic support or balloon pump support. The first successful LVAD implantation as a BTT occurred in 1985.[10] The first-generation LVAD was first approved by the Food and Drug Administration (FDA) for BTT in 1994. Since then, the second-generation and third-generation LVADs have largely superseded the original devices. The landmark REMATCH trial has resulted in FDA approval of LVADs for DT because the study proved clinically meaningful survival benefit as well as improved quality of life as compared with medical therapy alone.[4]

There has been significant progress in the design of LVADs. First-generation devices were large and designed to deliver pulsatile circulation. There were complex designs with significant moving parts, which impacted durability. The size of the first-generation devices necessitated placement in the preperitoneal space or intraperitoneal space.[10] Despite their successes, there were very high infection rates associated with these devices, in addition to the many mechanical problems related to the number of mechanical parts.

Devices have since progressed to a third generation of devices, which deliver continuous axial circulation rather than pulsatile circulation. They are typically smaller and deliver axial flow pumps requiring a smaller conduit of power with less moving components. These devices are associated with a lower rate of infection when compared with the first-generation devices.[2,11,12] The HeartMate 3 (St. Jude Medical - St. Paul Tech Center, MN, USA) was approved by the FDA in August 2017 for patients with NYHA class IIIb and class IV heart failure. These newer devices now represent greater than 90% of LVAD implanted.[2,3] In addition, the continuous improvement in surgical repertoires contributes to the continued improvement in infection rates.

SURVIVAL

With the progress in LVAD designs, clinical management, and improved surgical techniques, survival with LVAD continues to increase. With current continuous flow devices, the survival rate at 1 and 2 years is at 80% and 70%,[2] respectively.

Infection remains a major cause of morbidity and mortality in LVAD patients.[13,14] In the 1980s, with early mechanical devices, 80% of all device-related mortality were due to infection with subsequent progress in reduction of infection rates.[15] Currently, reports of infection-related adverse events largely come from 3 large multicenter registries for mechanical assist devices: (1) the Interagency Registry for Mechanically Assisted Circulatory Support (INTERMACS), the North American registry; (2) the European Registry for Patients with Mechanical Circulatory Support (EUROMACS), the European registry; and (3) the International Society for Heart and Lung Transplant (ISHLT) Registry for Mechanically Assisted Circulatory Support (IMACS), which is the largest and only international registry.

The seventh INTERMACS report included at total of more than 15,000 patients who received a primary implant from June 2006 to December 2014.[2] In this report, infection was the fourth most common cause of death within 1 year of transplant (8.8%), following neurologic complications, multisystem organ failure, and withdrawal of support. It is uncertain, although possible, that infections may also have contributed to multisystem organ failure cases or withdrawal of support cases, which could represent higher rates of infection contributing to death in patients with LVADs.

Similarly, the first EUROMACS report described infection as the most common adverse event (35.3% of all report adverse events) and second most common cause of death (69 out of 293, 23.5%) in a cohort of 741 patients.[3]

DEFINITION

In 2010, the ISHLT defined infections related to LVADs to improve clinical-investigator communication between different centers. A set-standard definition permits analysis of the source and pathophysiology of LVAD infections in addition to guiding diagnosis and management of LVAD infections. Before these standardized definitions, the diagnosis of LVAD infections was difficult and resulted in the lack of consistent reporting in LVAD infections. Infections related to LVADs are separated into 3 categories: VAD-specific infections, VAD-related infections, and non-VAD-related infections,[16] as listed in **Boxes 1** and **2**; **Fig. 1** provides a visual illustration of these definitions.

VAD specific infections are defined as hardware-related infections and can involve the pump, cannula, pocket, or drive-line (DL) sites. Diagnosis of a VAD-specific infection is based on the fulfillment of major and minor clinical criteria for each specific type of infection. Criteria for diagnosis of a VAD-specific infection involve clinical, microbiological, histopathological, and radiological components. The major and minor criteria for pump or cannula infections and pocket infections are listed in **Boxes 3** and **4**. Subsequently, infections are deemed to be proven, probable, and possible or refuted depending on the fulfillment of these criteria. The original ISHLT consensus paper has further detailed diagnostic criteria of VAD-specific and VAD-related infections, which is not included in this article.[16]

Box 1
Classification of infections in patients using ventricular assist devices

VAD-specific infections

- Pump and/or cannula infections

- Pocket infections

- Driveline infections
  - Superficial infection
  - Deep infection

VAD-related infections

- Infective endocarditis

- BSIs (including CVC-associated BSIs)
  CVC present
  - Bloodstream infection presumed VAD related
  - Bloodstream infection presumed CVC related
  No CVC present
  - Bloodstream infection VAD related
  - Bloodstream infection non-VAD related

- Mediastinitis
  - VAD related
    - Sternal wound infection surgical site infection-organ space
    - Pocket infection (continuous with mediastinum or already situated in the mediastinum depending on the device used)
  - Non-VAD related
    - Other causes of mediastinitis, perforation of the esophagus

Non-VAD infections

- Lower respiratory tract infection

- Cholecystitis

- *Clostridium difficile* infection

- Urinary tract infection

Abbreviation: CVC, central venous catheter.

> **Box 2**
> **Recommended international definitions for nonventricular assist device infections for registry data gathering**
>
> - Lower respiratory tract infections[a]
> - Cholecystitis[a]
> - C difficile infection[b]
> - Urinary tract infection[a]
>
> [a] Defined as per Centers for Disease Control and Prevention/National Healthcare Safety Network 30 definition.
> [b] Defined as per Health Protection Agency, UK definitions, and Infectious Disease Society of America definitions.

DL infections are the most commonly occurring infection in LVAD patients.[14,17–20] These infections may be a result of local trauma at the exit site and can occur either early or late. Goldstein and colleagues[18] showed 9.8% of all patients had an adverse event due to a DL infection. The mean time to develop first DL infection is 6.6 months. The only strong predictor of DL infections is age, with the younger patients at

> **Box 3**
> **Definition of terms used for the diagnosis of ventricular assist device–specific pump and/or cannula infection**
>
> *Major clinical criteria*
>
> - If the VAD is not removed, then an indistinguishable organism (genus, species, and antimicrobial susceptibility pattern) recovered from 2 or more peripheral blood cultures taken 12 hours apart with no other focus of infection or all of 3 or a majority of 4 separate positive blood cultures (with the first and last sample drawn at least 1 hour apart) with no other focus of infection.
>
> - When 2 or more positive blood cultures are taken from the CVC and peripherally at the same time and defined by criteria in **Box 4** as either BSI-VAD related or presumed VAD related
>
> - Echocardiogram positive for VAD-related IE (TEE recommended for patients with prosthetic valves, rated at least "possible IE" by clinical criteria, or complicated IE [paravalvular abscess] and in any patient in whom VAD-related infection is suspected and TTE is nondiagnostic; TTE as the first test in other patients) defined as follows: intracardiac mass suspected to be vegetation adjacent to or in the outflow cannula, or in an area of turbulent flow such as regurgitant jets, or consistent with a vegetation on implanted material, or abscess, or new partial dehiscence of outflow cannula
>
> *Minor clinical criteria*
>
> - Fever ≥38°C
>
> - Vascular phenomena, major arterial emboli, septic pulmonary infarcts, mycotic aneurysm, intracerebral or visceral, conjunctival hemorrhage, and Janeway lesions
>
> - Immunologic phenomena: glomerulonephritis, Osler nodes, Roth spot
>
> - Microbiologic evidence: positive blood culture that does not meet criteria as noted above (excluding single positive culture for coagulase-negative staphylococci, excluding *Staphylococcus lugdunensis*)
>
> *Abbreviations:* CVC, central venous cannula; TEE, transesophageal echocardiogram; TTE, transthoracic echocardiogram.

Box 4
Definition of terms used for the diagnosis of ventricular assist device–specific pocket infection

Major clinical criteria

- Microbiologic: aspirated fluid culture positive or fluid/pus diagnostic of infection
- Radiologic: new fluid collection by radiologic criteria: CT/US/Indium (enhancement or gas or sinus tract or leukocyte migration)

Minor clinical criteria

- Fever ≥38°C with no other recognized cause
- New local erythema over the pocket site
- Local pain and tenderness
- Induration or swelling
- Radiologic evidence: lymphangitis seen radiologically or
- New fluid collection without major criteria (above) and without diagnostic culture but not explained by other clinical conditions such as failure/anasarca/seroma

Abbreviation: US, ultrasound.

---

increased risk of DL infections. It was deduced that younger patients were likely to be more active, which puts them at higher risk of local trauma to the DL exit site.[19]

VAD-related infections include infective endocarditis (IE), bloodstream infection (BSI; both intravascular catheter-related and non-related), and mediastinitis. The definitions for these infections do not defer from the diagnostic criteria for these infections in non-VAD patients.

Non-VAD-related infections include all infections that are not directly attributed to the VAD but occur frequently in hospitalized and immunocompromised patients. Once again, these definitions do not defer from international definition of infections. The ISHLT has listed the most common non-VAD-related infections, and their recommended international definitions are listed in **Box 2**. A higher incidence of non-VAD infections in LVAD patients likely reflect that they have prolonged health care exposure and in addition frequently require invasive monitoring or therapy during their inpatient stay.

DIAGNOSIS

Presentation of LVAD infections can be varied and often can present as nonspecific symptoms. Localized symptoms can occur in superficial DL infections and should prompt patients to seek medical care. Deeper infection can present insidiously or acutely if bacteremia has occurred. An accurate history as well as a detailed physical examination, with a proper inspection of DL exit site, should be performed. The DL exit site should be examined for any evidence of trauma, local evidence of infection, or DL damage.[21]

Diagnosis is similar to other implantable cardiac device infections with a recommended minimum of 3 sets of blood cultures required in suspected cases of VAD-specific and VAD-related infections. The first and last culture ideally should be taken at least 1 hour apart, preferably from 2 separate peripheral sites, based on the Modified Duke's criteria.[22] In patients who are hemodynamically stable, consider at least 2 sets before the initiation of antimicrobials. In patients with central or peripheral venous access, 1 set should be taken from the catheter together with a set of peripheral blood cultures. A transesophageal or transthoracic echocardiogram is recommended to assess for vegetations or abscess formation.[16,19] A sterile aspirate for Gram staining as well as routine bacterial and fungal culture should be sent in the event pus is seen along the DL exit site.[14,16] Inflammatory markers (including C-reactive protein, erythrocyte sedimentation rate, and white cell count) are useful in assessing patients who may have an LVAD infection.[22–28]

If the LVAD or any significant part of the device was removed, detailed sampling of the device should be sent for Gram stain and routine bacterial and fungal culture. Any suspicious surrounding tissue should also be sent for histology, Gram stain, and bacterial and fungal culture.

In addition, imaging of the LVAD, including along the length of the DL, is often required with ultrasound or computed tomography (CT) imaging if a pocket or deep DL infection is suspected.[29,30] CT or ultrasound imaging can be useful in guiding aspiration of collections around the device for diagnostic purposes. There have been studies to suggest the use of PET with fluoro-D-glucose integrated CT for the diagnosis of LVAD-associated infections.[31–34] Another article describes the use of integrated leukocyte planar scintigraphy with CT for diagnosis.[35] However, no specific modality has been proven to definitively exclude a deep-tissue space infection on its own.[29]

Part of the workup should include an assessment for non-VAD-related infections, and any relevant investigations carried out.

MICROBIOLOGY

Bacterial pathogens remain the dominant cause of infections in LVAD infections. As with other prosthetic devices, the most common bacteria are gram-positive bacterium that colonizes the skin and can adhere to implanted material and form biofilms. *Staphylococcus aureus* and *Staphylococcus epidermidis* cause greater than 50% of infection, which is similar to infections in other implantable cardiac devices.[11,36–38] The most common gram-negative bacterium that cause LVAD infections is *P aeruginosa* followed by *Enterobacteriaceae* sp and *Serratia* sp.[36] Multi-drug-resistant organisms, such as methicillin-resistant *S aureus* (MRSA), vancomycin-resistant Enterococcus, and carbapenem-resistant Enterobacteriaceae, can be difficult to treat effectively, and screening for these organisms should be carried out before implant and throughout the patient's hospitalization.

Fungal infections are less common and account for only 7.4% in an IMACS report for 2013 to 2015.[39] Most fungal infections are non-VAD-related pneumonia/pulmonary infection, non-VAD-related BSI, and non-VAD-related urinary tract infection.[39] VAD-specific and VAD-related fungal infections only account for 0.37% and 0.53% of all patients in the registry. The report also suggested that fungal infections are more likely to occur early rather than late (<3 months vs >3 months after implantation). *Candida* species are the most common pathogen in fungal infections.[40–43] *Aspergillus* sp have also been reported in cases of LVAD infections, with high mortalities.[43–45]

It is important for clinicians to be aware of the local resistance patterns in both gram-positive and gram-negative infections in their hospitals. Clinicians are advised to be guided by local antimicrobial guidelines for antibiotic prescription in both suspected and confirmed LVAD associated infections.

PRINCIPLES OF MANAGEMENT

The principles of management largely rely on observational data and expert opinion in the field. As such, the management of VAD-specific and VAD-related infections is highly individualized, and the input of an infection specialist who is familiar with such devices should be obtained in most cases.

In patients with a suspected superficial DL infection without systemic illness or sepsis, there could be consideration for ambulatory management. If VAD-specific infections, including deep DL infection, is suspected or if the patient has any clinical evidence of sepsis, the patient should be managed in the inpatient setting.[46]

There should be emphasis on obtaining the identification of the causative pathogen in all cases to guide the appropriate choice of antimicrobials. Although superficial DL infections can be managed conservatively, in deep tissue infections, early surgical input is important should debridement be required. Surgical management may range from local debridement to DL site change to deep surgical drainage and vacuum-assisted closure system.[47,48]

Initial empiric treatment should be guided by local epidemiology and local antimicrobial guidelines. However, empiric treatment should typically include antimicrobials targeting Staphylococcus sp and Pseudomonas sp. Antibiotics should subsequently be tailored to specific organisms obtained from relevant specimens. The length of intravenous and oral antibiotics should be guided by an infection specialist. Therapeutic drug monitoring is recommended where available for antimicrobials (eg, vancomycin, voriconazole, posaconazole, aminoglycosides) to ensure optimum and safe treatment. Close monitoring of the international normalized ratio (INR) is usually required because antimicrobials potentially affect the INR.[46]

Recurrent or relapsed infections pose a difficult challenge in LVAD infections. There is limited literature available regarding the incidence, prevalence, and consensus definition of relapsed or recurrent infections. A combination of medical and surgical intervention is recommended, including intravenous and long-term suppressive antibiotics, surgical drainage, surgical debridement, or device exchange.

In many centers, patients who get serious LVAD infections are expedited to the urgent transplant waiting list. In patients who manage to get a heart transplant, the removal of the LVAD allows complete cure of the initial infection. However, the input of an infection specialist is necessary around the time of transplant and removal of the LVAD as well as for follow-up after transplant.[20,49,50] Patients should be stable on antimicrobial treatment at the time of heart transplant.

Key summary points for VAD-specific and VAD-related infections are found in later discussion.

MANAGEMENT OF VENTRICULAR ASSIST DEVICE–SPECIFIC INFECTIONS

It is important to determine whether an infection involving the LVAD components are superficial or deep. Superficial DL or pocket infections may successfully be treated without any surgical intervention, whereas a deep DL or pocket infection may require surgical debridement. The principles of treatment of VAD-specific infection should be similar to other cardiovascular implantable devices.[51,52]

For superficial pocket or DL infections, treatment with intravenous or oral antibiotics for a minimum of 2 weeks until satisfactory clinical resolution of the infection is recommended (eg, resolution of erythema or tenderness over DL exit site).[19,46] The principles of management as described above should be followed, with every effort made to identify the causative organism. In superficial DLIs, a reemphasis of DL immobilization and DL care should be given to the patient and carer.[46]

Deep pocket or deep DL infections should be managed as deep infections similar to other cardiac devices with a recommendation of 6 weeks of antibiotics, initially started intravenously.[19,46] Consider early surgical review where a deep infection is suspected.

In the case of a deep DL infection, transfer of the DL exit site to a location away from the previous infection may be recommended. In many cases, the use of long-term suppressive antimicrobials would be warranted, but the decision should be made together with an infection expert.[19,46,50,53,54] DL infections of unknown depth should be assessed clinically and may require treatment as a deep DL infection. Despite the use of suppressive antimicrobials, relapse remains common.[55,56]

Pump or cannula infections can pose a major clinical problem because curative treatment may be difficult without LVAD removal. The management plan would be determined by the goal of LVAD in the individual patient. Surgical drainage and debridement may be warranted for source control and should be considered for all patients. In BTT patients, antimicrobials would typically be continued until heart transplantation.[46] Intravenous antimicrobials should be initiated at the start, and depending on the organism isolated and clinical progress, an oral switch may be possible. Duration of treatment after device explant and heart transplant should be guided by an infection specialist. In DT patients, the use of 6 weeks of intravenous antimicrobials followed by further oral antimicrobials may be warranted. Long-term suppressive oral antimicrobials would usually be warranted.[46] An infection specialist opinion would be essential in such cases.

LVAD replacement may be needed in cases of the following: (1) persistent bacteremia and sepsis despite optimal targeted antibiotics; (2) relapsing or recurring infections; (3) septic emboli despite optimal targeted antibiotics.[55–57] For DT patients, LVAD replacement may be the only option for complete cure of the infection.[55,58,59] The authors acknowledge the decision and timing of replacement of LVAD can be difficult because patients are dependent on the LVAD and are potentially critically ill.

MANAGEMENT OF VENTRICULAR ASSIST DEVICE–RELATED INFECTIONS

In catheter-related bloodstream infections (CRBSI), removal of the central catheter is key in management. The guidelines from the Infectious Disease Society of America are recommended for CRBSI.[60] *Staphylococcus* sp infections may be problematic because of the propensity to bind to prosthetic material and form biofilms, and seeding of the LVAD should be considered.[61–63] In non-CRBSI, source finding of the bacteremia should be a key priority. If the bloodstream infection can be attributed to a specific source (eg, urinary tract infection) and seeding of the prosthetic material can be reasonably ruled out, the patient may be able to avoid prolonged antimicrobials of 6 weeks. If no specific source is found, the VAD pump or cannula infection should be suspected, and advised treatment length should be for a minimum of 6 weeks.[46]

In the cases of mediastinitis in LVAD patients, prolonged antimicrobial therapy for a minimum of 6 weeks is usually required. Surgical debridement is often indicated.

IE in LVAD patients may require ≥6 weeks of antimicrobials depending on the causative organisms and the clinical response to treatment. A surgical approach may be required, and treatment is similar to a pump or pocket infection. As with pump or pocket infections, suppressive oral antimicrobials would be warranted in cases where LVAD explant is not possible.

PREVENTION

In view of the significant morbidity and mortality associated with LVAD infections, prevention of LVAD infections should be an important component in all programs that insert LVADs. A comprehensive infection prevention and control program should be detailed in each center with an emphasis on decolonization, prophylactic antibiotics, nosocomial and catheter-related devices, perioperative management, and postoperative management for each patient undergoing LVAD insertion. The ISHLT consensus document has precise details of each component, and the authors have summarized some of the general recommendations here.[46]

General considerations include avoiding implantation of LVADs in the setting of suspected infection. The authors recommend the input of an infection specialist if an infection is suspected before implantation to ensure appropriate treatment is given. Routine investigations for patients with fevers or a high white cell count include blood and urine cultures, a urinalysis, and a chest radiograph. Further investigations are dependent on the clinical presentation.

It is recommended all patients undergoing LVAD insertion should be screened for S aureus in their nose and groin.[63] Patients who are colonized with either methicillin-sensitive S aureus or MRSA should have preoperative bathing with antiseptic soap and the use of mupirocin nasal decontamination in the patient with nasal carriage, which is shown to reduce S aureus infections.[64–66]

The perioperative and intraoperative management is important during implantation of LVADs. The ISHLT paper has specifically addressed several issues regarding perioperative and intraoperative management.[46] Although there are no specific randomized trials regarding antimicrobial prophylaxis (AP), consensus guidelines recommend the use of AP for all surgical patients, including cardiothoracic surgery. Local data should be used to guide the choice of antibiotic prophylaxis, but all regimens should always have Staphylococcus sp cover. In centers where MRSA rates are high, it is also recommended specific MRSA cover should be part of the AP regimen. ISHLT do not recommend routine use of gram-negative[67] or fungal prophylaxis.[68] Consensus agreement recommends initiation of antibiotics within 1 hour of skin incision. The recommended AP duration is 24 to 48 hours because AP beyond this introduces concern for the development of antimicrobial resistance without any impact on surgical-site infection rates.

DL immobilization early after surgery is a key component in preventing LVAD-associated infections because it remains one of the weaknesses in LVAD implantation. The DL remains one of the few components that is external. The goal is to minimize line movement, which is linked to local trauma of the DL and subsequent infections.[18,21,56,69,70]

The care of LVADs, particularly the DL exit site, should be emphasized with patients. It is recommended that a multidisciplinary team with thorough training in the management of LVAD should be involved in the management and care postoperatively. DL care and prevention of trauma of the DL exit site needs to be emphasized, because they are important risk factors to DL infections. It is recommended that continuous education to patients and caregivers be a key component in long-term management of LVAD.[71] Consideration should be given to education regarding dressing changes, personal hygiene, DL site immobilization, and other individual lifestyle factors. It should be emphasized that most DL infections occur after 3 months.[72]

With regards to dressing changes, an aseptic technique in accordance to local institutional policies should follow the postoperative period.[73] Daily changes are recommended with inspection until the DL exit site has fully healed. Once healed, dressing changes can be decreased to 1 to 3 times weekly. Patients or caregivers should be trained by a qualified health professional before discharge and competency regularly reviewed.[21] The DL exit site should be inspected at each clinic visit for local signs of infection or trauma.

SUMMARY

LVADs have changed the management of heart failure, and outcomes continue to improve because of progress in the design of the devices as well as improvement in the surgical repertoire and management of the devices. However, infections still contribute to a large proportion of morbidity and mortality in LVADs. A high index of suspicion should be maintained for infection in patients with LVAD. Early and aggressive medical and surgical treatment should be pursued in cases of LVAD-associated infections. A multidisciplinary team is key in the prevention of infections in LVAD, which should be involved in the perioperative, intraoperative, and postoperative periods of LVAD implantation.

DL infections still remain the most common infection. The ideal LVAD would be a fully implantable device without an external DL; maybe this will be developed in the future.

Despite improvement in the survival of patients that has resulted from better prevention and management strategies for LVAD infections, there remains the need for continued studies and surveillance data gathering to improve the understanding of these complex infections. The authors recommend for centers involved in LVAD implantation and management to actively participate in international registries, which will result in meaningful data analysis to guide future management of LVAD infections.

REFERENCES

1. Go AS, Mozaffarian D, Roger LR, et al. Heart disease and stroke statistics 2013 update. Circulation 2013;127(1):6–245.
2. Kirklin JK, Naftel D, Pagani F, et al. Seventh INTERMACS annual report: 15,000 patients and counting. J Heart Lung Transplant 2015;34(12):1495–504.
3. By TM, Mohacsi P, Gummert J, et al. The European Registry for Patients with Mechanical Circulatory Support (EUROMACS): first annual report. Eur J Cardiothorac Surg 2015;47(5):770–6.
4. Dembitsky WP, Tector AJ, Park S, et al. Left ventricular assist device performance with long-term circulatory support: lessons from the REMATCH trial. Ann Thorac Surg 2004;78:2123–9.
5. Aaronson KD, Slaughter MS, McGee E, et al. Evaluation of the Heartware HVAD left ventricular assist device system for the treatment of advanced heart failure: results of the ADVANCE bridge to transplant trial. Circulation 2010;122:2216.
6. Rose EA, Gelijins AC, Moskowitz AJ, et al. Long-term use of a ventricular assist device for end-stage heart failure. N Engl J Med 2001;345:1435–43.
7. Prichard R, Kershaw L, Goodall S, et al. Left ventricular device implantation impacts on hospitalisation rates, length of stay and out of hospital time. Heart Lung Circ 2018;27(6):708–15.
8. Health Quality Ontario. Left ventricular assist devices for destination therapy: a health technology assessment. Ont Health Technol Assess Ser 2016;16(3):1–60.
9. Tsiouris A, Paone G, Nemah HW. Short and long-term outcomes of 200 patients supported by continuous-flow left ventricular assist devices. World J Cardiol 2015;7(11):792–800.
10. Marcel R, Meyer DM. An overview of approved and investigational left ventricular assist devices. Proc (Bayl Univ Med Cent) 2004;17(4):407–10.
11. Slaughter MS, Rogers JG, Milano CA, et al. Advanced heart failure treated with continuous-flow left ventricular assist device. N Engl J Med 2009;361:2241–51.
12. Starling RC, Naka Y, Boyle AJ, et al. Results of the post-U.S. Food and Drug Administration-approval study with a continuous flow left ventricular assist device

as a bridge to heart transplantation: a prospective study using the INTERMACS. J Am Coll Cardiol 2011;57:1890–8.

13. Raju S, MacIver J, Foroutan F, et al. Long-term use of left ventricular assist devices: a report on clinical outcomes. Can J Surg 2017;60(4):236–46.

14. Trachtenberg B, Cordero-Reyes A, Elias B, et al. A review of infections in patients with left ventricular assist devices: prevention, diagnosis and management. Methodist Debakey Cardiovasc J 2015;11(1):28–32.

15. Zimpfer D, Netuka I, Schimitto JD, et al. Multicentre clinical trial experience with the HeartMate 3 left ventricular assist device: 30-day outcomes. Eur J Cardiothorac Surg 2016;50(3):548–54.

16. Hannan M, Husain S, Mattner F, et al. Working formulation for the standardization of definitions of infections in patients using ventricular assist devices. J Heart Lung Transplant 2011;30(4):375–84.

17. Leuck AM. Left ventricular assist device drive line infections: recent advances and future goals. J Thorac Dis 2015;7(12):2151–7.

18. Goldstein DJ, Naftel D, Holman W, et al. Continuous-flow devices and percutaneous site infections: clinical outcomes. J Heart Lung Transplant 2012;31(11):1151–7.

19. Nienaber JJ, Kusne S, Riaz T, et al. Clinical manifestations and management of left ventricular assist device-associated infections. Clin Infect Dis 2013;57(10): 1438–48.

20. Tong MZ, Smedira NG, Soltesz EG, et al. Outcomes of heart transplant after left ventricular assist device specific and related infection. Ann Thorac Surg 2015; 100:1292–7.

21. Feldman D, Pamboukian SV, Teuteberg JJ, et al. The 2013 International Society for Heart and Lung Transplantation guidelines for mechanical circulatory support: executive summary. J Heart Lung Transplant 2013;32:157–87.

22. Li JS, Sexton DJ, Mick N, et al. Proposed modifications to the Duke criteria for the diagnosis of infective endocarditis. Clin Infect Dis 2000;30:633–8.

23. Lennerz C, Vrazic H, Haller B, et al. Biomarker-based diagnosis of pacemaker and implantable cardioverter defibrillator pocket infections: a prospective, multi-centre, case-control evaluation. PLoS One 2017;12(3):e0172384.

24. Coakley G, Mathews C, Field M, et al. BSR & BHPR, BOA, RCGP and BSAC guidelines for management of the hot swollen joint in adults. Rheumatology (Oxford) 2006;45:1039–41.

25. Moran E, Byren I, Atkins BL. The diagnosis and management of prosthetic joint infections. J Antimicrob Chemother 2010;65(Suppl 3):iii45–54.

26. Muller M, Morawietz L, Hasart O, et al. Diagnosis of periprosthetic infection following total hip arthroplasty—evaluation of the diagnostic values of pre- and intraoperative parameters and the associated strategy to preoperatively select patients with a high probability of joint infection. J Orthop Surg Res 2008;3:31.

27. Klug D, Lacroix D, Savoye C, et al. Systemic infection related to endocarditis on pacemaker leads: clinical presentation and management. Circulation 1997;95: 2098–107.

28. Schuhmann MU, Ostrowski KR, Draper EJ, et al. The value of C-reactive protein in the management of shunt infections. J Neurosurg 2005;103(3 suppl):223–30.

29. Carr CM, Jacob J, Park SJ, et al. CT of left ventricular assist devices. Radiographics 2010;30:429–44.

30. Schroff GS, Ocazionez D, Akkanti B, et al. CT imaging of complications associated with continuous-flow left ventricular assist devices (LVADs). Semin Ultrasound CT MR 2017;38(6):616–28.

31. Dejust S, Guedec-Ghelfi R, Blanc-Autrant E, et al. Infection of ventricular assist device detected and monitored by 18F-FDG PET/CT. Clin Nucl Med 2017; 42(9):695–6.

32. Tlili G, Picard F, Pinaquy JB, et al. The usefulness of FDG PET/CT imaging in suspicion of LVAD infection. J Nucl Cardiol 2014;21(4):845–8.

33. Kim J, Feller ED, Chen W, et al. FDG PET/CT imaging for LVAD associated infections. JACC Cardiovasc Imaging 2014;7(8):839–42.

34. Avramovic N, Dell'Aquilla AM, Weckesser M. Metabolic volume performs better than SUVmax in the detection of left ventricular assist device driveline infection. Eur J Nucl Med Mol Imaging 2017;44(11):1870–7.

35. Maniar S, Kondareddy S, Topkara V. Left ventricular assist device-related infections: past, present and future. Expert Rev Med Devices 2011;8(5):627–34.

36. Gordon SM, Schmitt SK, Jacobs M, et al. Nosocomial bloodstream infections in patients with implantable left ventricular assist devices. Ann Thorac Surg 2001; 72:725–30.

37. Hussain AA, Baghdy Y, Wazni OM, et al. Microbiology of cardiac implantable electronic device infections. JACC Clin Electrophysiol 2016;2(4):498–505.

38. Fukunaga M, Goya M, Nagashima M, et al. Identification of causative organism in cardiac implantable electronic device infections. J Cardiol 2017;70(5):411–5.

39. Morrisey O, Xie R, Schaenmann J, et al. Epidemiology of Fungal Infections (FI) in Mechanical Circulatory Support Device (MCSD) recipients: analysis of IMACS registry 2013-2015. J Heart Lung Transpl 2017;36(4):S27.

40. Aslam S, Hernandez M, Thornby J, et al. Rish factors and outcomes of fungal ventricular-assist device infections. Clin Infect Dis 2010;50:664–71.

41. Shoham S, Shaffer R, Sweet L, et al. Fungal left ventricular assist device endocarditis. Ann Thorac Surg 2001;71:614–8.

42. Bagdasarian NG, Malani AN, Pagani FD, et al. Fungemia associated with left ventricular assist device support. J Card Surg 2009;24:763–5.

43. Bagdasarian NG, Duggan JM. Left ventricular assist device infections: three case reports and a review of the literature. ASAIO J 2002;48:2–7.

44. Maly J, Szarszoi O, Dorazilova Z, et al. Case report: atypical fungal obstruction of the left ventricular assist device outflow cannula. J Cardiothorac Surg 2014;9:40.

45. Barbone A, Pini D, Gross P, et al. Aspergillus left ventricular assist device endocarditis. Ital Heart J 2004;5(11):876–80.

46. Kusne S, Mooney M, Danziger-Isakov L, et al. An ISHLT consensus document for prevention and management strategies for mechanical circulatory support infection. J Heart Lung Transplant 2017;36(10):1137–53.

47. Baradarian S, Stahovich M, Krause S, et al. Case series: clinical management of persistent mechanical assist device drive line drainage using vacuum-assisted closure therapy. ASAIO J 2006;52:354–6.

48. Kouretas PC, Burch PT, Kaza AK, et al. Management of deep wound complications with vacuum-assisted therapy after Berlin Heart EXCOR ventricular assist device placement in the pediatric population. Artif Organs 2009;33:922–5.

49. Koval CE, Thuita L, Moazami N, et al. Evolution and impact of drive-line infection in a large cohort of continuous-flow ventricular assist device recipients. J Heart Lung Transpl 2014;33(11):1164–72.

50. Schulman AR, Martens TP, Russo MJ, et al. Effect of left ventricular assist device infection on post-transplant outcomes. J Heart Lung Transplant 2009;28(3): 237–42.

51. Sandoe JA, Barlow G, Chambers JB, et al. Guidelines for the diagnosis, prevention and management of implantable cardiac electronic device infection. Report of a

joint Working Party project on behalf of the British Society for Antimicrobial Chemotherapy (BSAC, host organization), British Heart Rhythm Society (BHRS), British Cardiovascular Society (BCS), British Heart Valve Society (BHVS) and British Society for Echocardiography (BSE). J Antimicrob Chemother 2015;70(2):325–59.

52. Baddour LM, Epstein AE, Erickson CC, et al. Update on cardiovascular implantable electronic device infections and their management: a scientific statement from the American Heart Association. Circulation 2010;121(3):458–77.

53. Haddad E, Lescure FX, Ghodhbane W, et al. Left ventricular assist pump pocket infection: conservative treatment strategy for destination therapy candidates. Int J Artif Organs 2017;40(3):90–5.

54. Jennings DL, Chopra A, Chambers R, et al. Clinical outcomes associated with chronic antimicrobial suppression therapy in patients with continuous-flow left ventricular assist devices. Artif Organs 2014;38:875–9.

55. Levy DT, Guo Y, Simkins J, et al. Left ventricular assist device exchange for persistent infection: a case series and review of the literature. Transpl Infect Dis 2014;16:453–60.

56. Zierer A, Melby S, Voellar RK, et al. Late-onset driveline infections: the Achilles' heel of prolonged left ventricular assist device support. Ann Thorac Surg 2007; 84(2):515–20.

57. Toda K, Yonemoto Y, Fujita T, et al. Risk analysis of bloodstream infection during long-term left ventricular assist device support. Ann Thorac Surg 2012;94: 1387–93.

58. Chamogeorgakis T, Koval CE, Smedira NG, et al. Outcomes associated with surgical management of infections related to the HeartMate II left ventricular assist device: Implications for destination therapy patients. J Heart Lung Transplant 2012;31(8):904–6.

59. Abicht T, Gordon R, Meehan K, et al. Complex HeartMate II infection treated with pump exchange to HeartWare HVAD. ASAIO J 2013;59:188–92.

60. Leonard AM, Allon M, Bouza E, et al. Clinical practice guidelines for the diagnosis and management of intravascular catheter-related infection: 2009 update by the Infectious Diseases Society of America. IDSA guidelines. Available at: http://www.idsociety.org/Guidelines/Patient_Care/IDSA_Practice_Guidelines/Other_Guidelines/Other/Management_of_Catheter-related_Infections. Accessed January 15, 2018.

61. Toba AF, Akashi H, Arrecubieta C, et al. Role of biofilm in staphylococcus aureus and staphylococcus epidermidis ventricular assist device driveline infections. J Thorac Cardiovasc Surg 2011;141(5):1259–64.

62. Römling U, Balsalobre C. Biofilm infections, their resilience to therapy and innovative treatment strategies. J Intern Med 2012;272(6):541–61.

63. Kusne S, Danziger-Isakov L, Mooney M, et al. Infection control and prevention practices for mechanical circulatory support: an international survery. J Heart Lung Transplant 2013;32:484.

64. Kallen AJ, Wilson CT, Larson RJ. Perioperative intranasal mupirocin for the prevention of surgical-site infections: systematic review of the literature and meta-analysis. Infect Control Hosp Epidemiol 2005;26(12):916–22.

65. Herbert C, Robicsek A. Decolonization therapy in infection control. Curr Opin Infect Dis 2010;23:340–5.

66. Climo MW, Yokoe DS, Warren DK, et al. Effect of daily chlorhexidine bathing on hospital-acquired infection. N Engl J Med 2013;368:962–72.

67. Bratzler DW, Dellinger EP, Olsen KM, et al. Clinical practice guidelines for antimicrobial prophylaxis in surgery. Am J Health Syst Pharm 2013;70:195–283.

68. Husain S, Sole A, Alexander BD, et al. The 2015 International Society for Heart and Lung Transplantation guidelines for the management of fungal infections in mechanical circulatory support and cardiothoracic organ transplant recipients: executive summary. J Heart Lung Transplant 2016;35:261–82.
69. Sharma V, Deo SV, Stulak JM, et al. Driveline infections in left ventricular assist devices: implications for destination therapy. Ann Thorac Surg 2012;84:1381–6.
70. Yarboro LT. Technique for minimizing and treating driveline infections. Ann Thorac Surg 2014;3:557–62.
71. Barber J, Leslie G. A simple education tool for ventricular assist device patients and their caregivers. J Cardiovasc Nurs 2014;30:E1–10.
72. John R, Aaronson KD, Pae WE, et al. Drive-line infections and sepsis in patients receiving the HVAD system as a left ventricular assist device. J Heart Lung Transplant 2014;33(10):1066–73.
73. Cannon A, Elliott T, Ballew C, et al. Variability in infection control measures for the percutaneous lead among programs implanting long-term ventricular assist devices in the United States. Prog Transplant 2012;22:351–9.

Prosthetic Joint Infection Update

Elena Beam, MD[a,*], Douglas Osmon, MD[b]

KEYWORDS

- Prosthetic joint infection • Prevention • Biofilm • Sonicate fluid • Suppression

KEY POINTS

- Diagnosis of prosthetic joint infection (PJI) is established via a combination of preoperative and intraoperative tests.
- Treatment of PJI is individualized based on patient factors, microbiology, and surgical expertise.
- PJI presentation differs based on time from arthroplasty, with virulent organisms seen more commonly in early PJI.

INTRODUCTION/BACKGROUND

Total joint arthroplasties are increasing in the total number of procedures performed yearly given excellent functional improvement for the patient, and improvement in overall quality of life and pain relief the procedure provides. In the United States, the most commonly performed arthroplasty is a total knee arthroplasty (TKA), followed by total hip arthroplasty (THA), and more than 1 million of these combined are done annually in the United States.[1] The prevalence rates of THA and TKA in 2010 were estimated at 0.83% and 1.52%, respectively, of the population in the United States.[1] The annual number of arthroplasties is expected to increase to 3.48 million by 2030.[2] The numbers for THA performed annually are lower in the United States; however, the same uptrend in the total number of procedures is expected over the coming years. Similarly, increasing numbers of patient are expected to undergo other total joint replacements, including shoulder, elbow, and ankle. A majority of arthroplasties currently performed are for a primary indication of osteoarthritis-related complications.

EPIDEMIOLOGY

The overall risk of developing prosthetic joint infection (PJI) depends on several modifiable and nonmodifiable factors. Historical rates of PJI showed a highest risk period

[a] Division of Infectious Disease, Department of Internal Medicine, Mayo Clinic, 200 First Street Southwest, Rochester, MN 55905, USA; [b] Division of Infectious Disease, Departments of Medicine and Orthopedic Surgery, Mayo Clinic, 200 First Street Southwest, Rochester, MN 55905, USA
* Corresponding author.
E-mail address: beam.elena@mayo.edu

Infect Dis Clin N Am 32 (2018) 843–859
https://doi.org/10.1016/j.idc.2018.06.005
0891-5520/18/© 2018 Elsevier Inc. All rights reserved.

id.theclinics.com

during the first 2 years after the arthroplasty procedure, theoretically while there is ongoing soft tissue healing and postoperative inflammation still present. After a primary hip or knee arthroplasty, a cumulative incidence of 0.5% after the first year and 1.4% after 10 years has been reported, accounting for approximately 1.5 infections per 1000 person-joint-years.[3] More importantly PJI is the most common cause of TKA failure; for example, in a large study of 11,134 total knee arthroplasties, the cumulative incidence of revision at 15 years was 6.1%, with 2.0% of the 6.1% done for PJI, whereas aseptic loosening was the second most common reason for revision and accounted for another 1.2%.[4] PJI is the third most common indication for revision hip arthroplasties.[2] The higher rate of PJIs in knee arthroplasties is expected to be secondary to less protective soft tissue coverage as well as higher stress in terms of mobility in the joint and soft tissue. Only smaller studies are available to guide the risk of PJI after shoulder and elbow arthroplasty. The risk of shoulder arthroplasty infection seems less than or similar to the risks of hip and knee surgery, although a higher rate of PJIs were reported complicating elbow arthroplasty, in up to 3.3% of the cases.[5]

SURGICAL FACTORS

Surgery-related risk factors for PJI include the location of arthroplasty, whether primary or revision surgery is performed, potential for soft tissue healing or soft tissue–related complications, and finally the potential for presence of subclinical infection at the time of prosthetic joint arthroplasty as related to prior infection of the joint.[6]

It is unclear whether the surgical approach or use of cemented or noncemented arthroplasty plays a role and the risk of PJI.[7] Additional surgery-related risks includes the use of metal-to-metal hinged prosthesis.[8] Postoperative complications, including postoperative hematoma and wound dehiscence, are additional factors.[9] Duration of surgical procedure has also been associated with an increased risk.[10] Postoperative myocardial infarction and atrial fibrillation are associated with a higher risk, likely secondary to the need for anticoagulation and antiplatelet use and potential bleeding complications from these.[9] Postoperative need for blood transfusion (not autologous) has been associated with PJI[9]; however, most recent surgical site infection (SSI) prevention guidelines recommend against withholding blood transfusion if required postoperatively in joint arthroplasty cases as a way to attempt to decrease risk of PJI.[11]

Additional potential modifiable risk factors are outlined in the SSI prevention guidelines. These include monitoring and prevention of perioperative hyperglycemia (blood glucose target <200 mg/dL), which is a known risk factor for SSI in other types of surgery.[11,12] The guidelines also recommend use of antimicrobial or nonantimicrobial soap preoperatively for bathing and use of appropriate type and timing of antimicrobial prophylaxis. Alcohol-based skin preparation in the operating room is also recommended, and perioperative normothermia should be maintained.

PATIENT FACTORS

Patient-specific factors that have been identified as increasing the rate of PJI include the presence of comorbidities, such as rheumatoid arthritis, diabetes mellitus, malignancy, chronic kidney disease, and sometimes obesity.[9,13] Additional patient-specific factors to consider include history and presence of lymphedema, immunosuppression, and history of difficult wound healing. Smoking and use of medications that may have an impact on wound healing potential, such as methotrexate, prednisone, or tumor necrosis factor α inhibitors and other biologic disease-modifying antirheumatic drugs, have been implicated in increased PJI risk. The American College of

Rheumatology has recently issued guidelines for management of antirheumatic medications for patients undergoing either elective THA or TKA, suggesting biologic medications be withheld 1 dosing cycle prior to the elective arthroplasty.[14]

History of infection, both present at the surgical site or other sites at the time of arthroplasty, raises the risk of PJI. Infection at other sites, particularly distant from the joint arthroplasty, likely increases the risk of PJI by seeding the joint with a transient bacteremia. Bloodstream infection in the setting of presence of a prosthetic joint is known risk factor for development of PJI, with the highest rate seen with staphylococcal bloodstream infections. Up to 25% to 34% of staphylococcal bloodstream infections in the presence of joint arthroplasty can become infected.[15,16] Although urinary tract infections seem to increase the rate of PJI, this is not shown in absence of symptoms, in the setting of asymptomatic bacteriuria.

The SSI prevention guidelines do not comment on preoperative staphylococcal decolonization; however, many studies support this approach and have noted decrease in PJI diagnoses after implementation of various decolonization protocols.[17] These have included universal decolonization as well as targeted decolonization of those identified as methicillin-sensitive *Staphylococcus aureus* or methicillin-resistant *S aureus* (MRSA) carriers preoperatively and generally use combination of chlorhexidine washes and mupirocin ointment in addition to modifying the perioperative intravenous (IV) antimicrobial use based on colonization findings. Various strategies have shown improvement in PJI rates and approaches are generally well tolerated. A major barrier to implementation of these practices is the involved coordination of care, in terms of testing (usually via a nasal swab), result follow-up, and implementation of appropriate action based on screening results, including use of mupiricon/chlorexidine and adjusting perioperative antimicrobial based on results.

Perioperative IV antimicrobial prophylaxis is optimized with the choice of antimicrobial based on spectrum of activity—primarily against skin flora, and administered at a time such that optimal antibiotic level is reached at tissue level at the time of incision, within an hour of incision.[18] Prophylaxis generally consists of a first-generation cephalosporin, such as cefazolin, and is preferred due to its bactericidal activity and quick administration.[18] Use of vancomycin is reserved for those with anaphylactic allergies or added in cases of known MRSA colonization. Those with a history of penicillin allergy identified at preoperative visit benefit from an allergy specialist and penicillin skin testing to confirm or remove the allergy from the list. In clean and clean-contaminated procedures, additional doses of prophylactic antimicrobial after incisions are closed is not routinely recommended, even in presences of a drain.[11]

HEALTH CARE COSTS/MORBIDITY AND MORTALITY

Each PJI diagnosis comes with significant morbidity to the patient as well as health care costs. The annual cost for infected revisions (through 2009) was $566 million and is expected to increase to $1.62 billion by 2020.[19] Some of the cost depends on the treatment approach, including debridement, antibiotics, and implant retention (DAIR) versus 1-stage exchange (OSE) compared with a 2-stage exchange (TSE), which generally requires at least 2 surgeries, and thus accounts for significant up-front costs. The antibiotic duration used after a TSE exchange is shorter compared with DAIR or OSE strategy—the relative monetary contribution is hard to predict because there is still some variance in the duration of antimicrobials administered after these surgeries.[19]

These infections require costs that are not directly related to surgery or antimicrobial therapy, which are harder to capture, including rehospitalization often followed by rehabilitation stays.

MICROBIOLOGY

Establishing a microbiologic diagnosis in PJI is key to providing the best treatment strategy, both in terms of surgical options as well as optimizing antimicrobial therapy to the most narrow and most active agent. The virulence of the organism and options of IV-directed antimicrobial therapy and oral antimicrobial therapy for longer-term suppression of the organism are factors that guide the overall surgical plan.

The microbiologic diagnosis, however, is challenging due to multiple factors, including biofilm formation, at the level of interaction of bacteria and prosthesis, and broad overall antimicrobial use, resulting in falsely negative cultures. Formation of biofilm is the major reason for inability to cure PJIs with antimicrobial therapy alone, without surgical intervention, to help address the biofilm formation. Even with surgical approach to PJI management, use of antibiofilm active agents remains of utmost importance, particularly in staphylococcal PJI.

Bacterial Causes

Many bacterial pathogens have been implicated in PJI; however, the most frequently seen pathogens are gram-positive cocci. S aureus and coagulase-negative staphylococci are the most common reported pathogens and tend to occur early postoperatively. Less frequent are gram-negative bacilli, polymicrobial infection, and anaerobic infection.

Factors that influence the microbiology include time from surgical intervention; soft tissue complications after surgery, including those related to wound healing, hematoma, and wound dehiscence; history of concomitant or preceding infection; previous known colonization with Staphylococcus and other drug-resistant organisms; and a patient's comorbidities, which may influence the type of infection noted.

Time to Infection

When evaluating potential microbiologic causes of PJI, it is helpful to evaluate the timeline from the arthroplasty procedure to development of infection. The timeline has an impact on the microbiologic differential diagnosis. **Table 1** includes the most common bacterial causes of PJI, broken down into early-onset, delayed-onset, and late-onset infections, and compares the different microbiology seen and approach to diagnosis based on time from joint arthroplasty. In general, early PJIs are defined as occurring within the first 3 months of initial surgery. The microbiologic differential of early PJI focuses on those bacterial pathogens that were introduced intraoperatively, with large bacterial burden or highly virulent organisms to account for the early presentation. As such, most common organisms include S aureus, higher relative proportion of anaerobic and aerobic gram-negative bacilli, and polymicrobial infections, along with coagulase-negative staphylococci. On the other hand, the delayed infection, although also most commonly still introduced at the time of original surgery or shortly thereafter, tends to present later, anywhere from 3 months to 1 year, with less virulent organisms. Polymicrobial infection and aerobic gram-negative bacteria become less common in these cases because these tend to be seen earlier. Finally, late-onset infections, typically defined as greater than 1 year or 2 years form arthroplasty, are usually a complication of different foci of infection and are a result of hematogenous seeding. Late-onset infections can to be caused by very indolent pathogens introduced the time of surgery; otherwise, these would have presented clinically earlier.

Arthroplasty Type

A second important factor to consider when approaching microbiologic differential diagnosis is the type and location of the joint arthroplasty. Shoulder arthroplasties,

Table 1
Description of prosthetic joint infection by time from arthroplasty

	Early Prosthetic Joint Infection	Delayed Onset (3–12 mo After Arthroplasty)	Late Onset
Synovial fluid			
White blood cell count (cells/μL)	>10,000	>3000	>3000
PMN (%)	>90	>80	>80
Serum CRP (mg/L)	>100[21]	>10	>10
Serum ESR (mm/h)	Not useful	>30	>30
Clinical presentation	Acute onset Wound drainage, fever, erythema, joint pain	Subacute joint pain; possible sinus tract formation, which diminishes pain	Systemic symptoms more likely with concomitant bacteremia, pain
Microbiologic differential	Virulent organisms *S aureus* Aerobic gram-negative bacilli Polymicrobial Anaerobic	Less virulent Coagulase-negative staphylococci *Enteroccus* *Cutibacterium*	*S aureus* β-Hemolytic streptococci Gram-negative bacilli
Etiology	Acquired during arthroplasty	Acquired during arthroplasty, early postoperatively	Hematogenous from other infectious focus
Histopathology	More than 5 PMNs per high-power field in 5 high-power fields		

Typical laboratory values derived from International Consensus definition.[20] Low virulence organism criteria could not be met, yet PJI still is present.

Data from Parvizi J, Gehrke T, International Consensus Group on Periprosthetic Joint Infection. Definition of periprosthetic joint infection. J Arthroplasty 2014;29(7):1331.

for example, have a particularly high incidence of infection due to *Cutibacterium* (previously *Propionibacterium*)—with *Cutibacterium acnes* the most common in shoulder arthroplasty infection, while being a much less common pathogen identified in other joint arthroplasty infections. This difference in rate of *Cutibacterium* infections is believed due exposure to the anaerobic bacteria, presumed to be at the time of initial arthroplasty procedure, given the proximity to the axilla, where the bacteria can be found normally. This consideration is important because it may have an impact on diagnostic treatment options. *Cutibacterium acnes*, a gram-positive anaerobic bacillus, may be difficult to isolate, if appropriate anaerobic cultures are not collected.

Fungal Infections

The most common fungal organisms leading to PJI are *Candida* species.[22] Overall, however, fungal organisms cause less than 1% of all PJIs. *Candida*, as a cause of monomicrobial PJI, is primarily seen in those with a history of revision arthroplasty, previous bacterial PJI, and previous exposure to antimicrobial use.[23] In addition, immunosuppression and diabetes are potential risk factors for development of *Candida* PJI.[23] *Candida albicans* is the most common candida species reported in the literature.[23,24] Even less frequent causes of fungal PJI are filamentous fungi and endemic dimorphic fungi—most of these are part of a disseminated infectious process that became complicated by PJI, typically from a primary pulmonary source.

Mycobacterial Infections

Mycobacteria represent a minority of PJIs. *Mycobacterium tuberculosis* complex, however, is on the differential in patients with history of previous active tuberculosis or history of latent tuberculosis. Diagnosis can be significantly delayed, by months or years after presentation.[25] Most cases of *Mycobacterium tuberculosis* PJI seem to occur in the setting of previous *Mycobacterium tuberculosis* infection of the native joint before the arthroplasty is placed, and in the wrist up to 31% has been reported in such case.[26]

Nontuberculous mycobacterial infections have also been rarely reported as a cause of PJI and limited to case reports and case series. These tend to have delayed diagnoses. In immunocompetent hosts, nontuberculous mycobacteria PJI are likely introduced intraoperatively; however, in immunocompromised hosts, this complication can arise from disseminated infectious process. Several case reports of PJI due to *Mycobacterium bovis* after intravesicular treatment with bacillus Calmette-Guérin (BCG) have also been recognized.[27,28]

Culture-negative Infections

Culture-negative PJIs are most commonly a result of previous antimicrobial exposure. As such, if microbiologic diagnosis is important for management, repeat testing off antimicrobial therapy, if possible, may be necessary. In addition to routine pathogens affected by previous antimicrobial treatment, culture-negative PJI can also be attributed to unusual and hard-to-culture types of organisms. These include a variety of rarely reported bacteria including *Coxiella burnetii* (causative agent of Q fever), *Brucella*, *Bartonella* and mycoplasma in addition to mycobacterial and fungal infections. All cases of PJI with negative aerobic/anaerobic bacterial cultures should have mycobacterial and fungal cultures performed. In addition to the hard-to-culture organisms as causative agents of culture negative PJI, it is possible that with improvement in the microbiologic techniques and use of broad-range polymerase chain reaction (PCR) and metagenomics shotgun sequencing, identifying novel causes of PJI will be possible.[29]

PREVENTION

Many strategies have been used over the years with an aim to decrease PJI after various types of procedures. The role of perioperative prevention strategies is reviewed previously in this article, in addition to a focus on optimizing any possible patient risk factors. Prevention of PJI after arthroplasty includes ongoing modification of patient factors.

Dental Prophylaxis

PJI prevention is changing. This is particularly true in regard to the recommendation of use of antibiotic prophylaxis with dental procedures and, similarly, use of antibiotic prophylaxis for urologic procedures in the presence of a prosthetic joint arthroplasty. Previous recommendations were based on the possibility that manipulation of tissue and potential bleeding complications with dental procedures (and other invasive procedures) could result in transient bacteremia, putting the prosthetic joint arthroplasty at risk. Thus, it was common practice to use antimicrobial prophylaxis in such cases. Studies have failed, however, to show an increased risk of PJI after such invasive dental procedures; furthermore, additional studies have failed to show any potential PJI reduction with use of antimicrobial prophylaxis.[30] In addition, a counterargument exists that such patients are likely faced with multiple transient bacteremias during the day that are associated with routine daily activities, and ongoing prophylaxis against all such activities is not realistic. Thus, based on currently available literature, the American Dental Association Council on Scientific Affairs recommends against the use of routine dental prophylaxis for PJI prevention.[31]

Use of antibiotic prophylaxis for dental procedures has been decreasing not only for PJI prevent but also for prevention of endocarditis.[32] The most recent guidelines from the American Academy of Orthopaedic Surgeons and American Dental Association were published in 2013 and suggested changing the longstanding practice of routine prophylactic antibiotics in this setting.[33] Maintenance of good oral hygiene was also recommended.[33]

Asymptomatic Bacteriuria Prophylaxis

Similarly, in context of higher risk of PJI in those with symptomatic urinary tract infections, previous practice extended to treat asymptomatic bacteriuria around the time of prosthetic joint arthroplasty surgery. More recent data, however, fail to support this practice; thus, in the absence of urinary tract symptoms, screening urinalysis and directed antibiotic therapy should not be routinely done.[34]

CLINICAL FEATURES

Clinical presentation of PJI can vary, depending on time from surgery, time from onset of symptoms, and antimicrobial use, in addition to the virulence of the organisms and whether a patient is immunocompromised.

Commonly reported symptoms include pain, warmth, and erythema at the joint site. Symptoms could also include fever, drainage, and wound dehiscence. If infection is complicated by bacteremia, systemic symptoms are to be expected. Infection that has broken through the soft tissue can result in a sinus tract formation, with direct communication with the underlying prosthesis. Patients tend to have less pain after sinus tract formation is noted. Among the reported symptoms, the most specific for diagnosis of PJI is formation of sinus tract, and the presence of sinus tract on its own can be considered definitive of a diagnosis of PJI. The most sensitive marker is likely pain, although this is nonspecific.

DIAGNOSIS

In general, in early PJIs, which occur as a result of perioperative contamination or difficulty with wound healing or postoperative hematoma formation, patients likely present with local signs and symptoms. Systemic symptoms may be present, however, if secondary bacteremia occurred.

The ideal diagnostic pathway to PJIs is to be able to identify all PJI cases, regardless of the bacterial pathogen type or load, previous antimicrobial exposure, presence of other inflammatory condition, or time from surgery, not at risk of potential contamination to potential contamination of the cultures. These factors, however, all pose a challenge to PJI diagnosis; many of the current diagnostic and supportive criteria rely on accuracy of the cultures as well as the inflammatory and immune response to infection and surgery.

There are several proposed diagnostic criteria for PJI. These include criteria endorsed by Infectious Diseases Society of America (IDSA), the Musculoskeletal Infection Society (MSIS), and the International Consensus Group on Periprosthetic Joint Infection, is a modification of the MSIS criteria.[20,35,36] These proposed criteria identify 2 groups, with definitive evidence of PJI as well as supportive evidence. A presence of sinus tract communicating with the prosthesis is common definitive criteria for presence of PJI among all the proposed definitions. Similarly, identification of same microorganism isolated from 2 or more cultures is considered definitive criteria. IDSA also defines evidence of purulence surrounding the prosthesis as definitive evidence of PJI. The supportive criteria by IDSA definition include presence of a single culture with virulent organism and presence of acute inflammation on histologic examination of periprosthetic tissue. MSIS criteria however, considers purulence surrounding the prosthesis to be supporting evidence of infection only, while International Consensus, have excluded purulence surrounding the prosthesis from the definitions altogether. The MSIS criteria include the following supporting evidence criteria: the presence of acute inflammation on histologic examination, single culture with any microorganisms, elevated synovial fluid leukocyte count, elevated synovial fluid neutrophil percentage, and elevated serum erythrocyte sedimentation rate (ESR) and CRP; at least 4 supporting criteria must be present for diagnosis of PJI.[36] The International Consensus criteria also consider the finding of ++ change on leukocyte esterase test strip of synovial fluid a supporting criteria.[20]

Inflammatory Markers

CRP and ESR are readily available peripheral blood tests with rapid turnaround time. They are the first diagnostic step in the setting of preoperative evaluation once a suspicion of PJI is raised by clinical signs and symptoms, in the absence of sinus tract formation, which in itself is diagnostic. This is particularly true for delayed-onset and late-onset infections. There is some limitation to use of these inflammatory markers with low virulent organisms, such as *Cutibacterium,* a common pathogen in shoulder PJI, where PJI can be present in the setting of normal inflammatory markers. Additional limitation of inflammatory markers is its use in the setting of other inflammatory conditions because these can lack specificity. **Table 1** includes the threshold values recommended by International Consensus for definition of PJI. CRP and ESR are impacted by postoperative inflammatory changes and thus are less useful during for diagnosis of acute PJI, however with a shorter half-life Of CRP, CRP is still included unlike ESR in early PJI definition.[36]

Synovial Fluid Testing

After inflammatory markers are obtained and there is ongoing suspicion of PJI, a diagnostic arthrocentesis should be performed to assess synovial fluid for cell count, polymorphonuclear cells (PMN), and synovial fluid culture. The results of the cell count and differential are unlikely to be impacted by antimicrobial therapy; however, the culture is affected with use of antimicrobial therapy in the preceding 2 weeks.[37] Microbiology can be supported by positive blood cultures if secondary bacteremia is present.

Cell Count and Differential

The supporting criteria in MSIS definition include synovial fluid analysis for total nucleated cell count and percentage of PMNs. The recommended diagnostic thresholds by International Consensus criteria are in **Table 1**, and these depend on the time from operative intervention. Although synovial fluid cell count greater than 3000 (cells/μL) and PMNs representing greater than 80% are recommended for delayed-onset and late-onset infections, the same numbers are not reliable in early postoperative course. During the early postoperative course, particularly within 6 weeks of surgery, there is expected normal inflammatory postsurgical response, and the recommended synovial fluid total nucleated cell count threshold is increased, at greater than 10,000 cells/μL, with greater than 90% PMNs. The threshold total nucleated cell count and PMN percentage are derived from studies that included primarily TKA and THA infections; thus, their use and appropriate threshold values for other joint arthroplasty, such as shoulder, elbow, and ankle arthroplasties, is not clear.[38,39]

Intraoperative Evaluation

Although gross purulence noted intraoperatively at the joint arthroplasty is considered diagnostic by the IDSA criteria for PJI, this was only considered supporting criteria by MSIS, given its subjective nature and other potential inflammatory causes of this appearance not related to infection.

Histopathology

Intraoperative evaluation can also include histopathologic samples, including frozen samples assessing for acute inflammation, which can help the orthopedic surgeon with a just-in-time decision on management of a patient. Early studies, however, showed low sensitivity of frozen section, and interpretation of this is likely biased by several factors.[40] Potential reasons for low sensitivity include infection due to low virulent pathogens (causing lower inflammatory changes), variability in expertise of the interpreting pathologist, and potential for sampling bias. Histologic findings are generally interpreted as positive for acute inflammation if greater than 5 neutrophils per high-power field in 5 high-power fields is noted.[20,41]

Periprosthetic Tissue Cultures and Sonicate Fluid Cultures

Greater than 3 and fewer than 6 deep cultures are recommended to be obtained the time of joint arthroplasty revision, if infection is suspected. Culture should include aerobic and anaerobic bacterial cultures routinely, with addition of fungal and mycobacterial cultures if those are suspected. Multiple culture specimens are necessary to help evaluate for potential contamination versus causative organisms seen in the culture results. A single culture due to a low virulence organism is generally considered a contaminant; however, if the same organism is seen in multiple cultures, a diagnosis of PJI can be made. Use of automated blood culture systems has improved both the sensitivity and specificity of routine bacterial cultures compared with previous use of agar plate cultures, an improvement suspected due to lower rate of contamination.[42]

   Although the use of sonicate fluid cultures is not likely necessary for routine cases, the sensitivity of sonicate fluid cultures is greater than routine periprosthetic tissue cultures, especially in those who received preoperative antimicrobial within 2 weeks of culture collection, and sonicate fluid cultures should be used in these cases. The explanation for increased sensitivity using sonicate fluid for culture is that the sonication is able to dislodge biofilm from the prosthesis, thereby increasing the ability to identify the bacterial pathogens.

IMAGING

Imaging studies add little value in diagnosis of PJI; however, they are useful in setting of a painful joint to explore alternative potential causes of pain and instability, such as fracture and dislocation. White blood cell tagged scans as well as PET scans are limited by increased activity within 12 months, due to postoperative inflammation.

NOVEL TESTS
Molecular Tests

Most recent studies have focused on molecular tests to increase the yield of identification of involved bacterial pathogen, including exploring previously culture-negative cases. These new methods also tend to have quick turnaround time.

Molecular methods have included use of broad-range 16S ribosomal RNA PCR and multiplex PCR panels (where identification of only the bacteria for which primers are included is possible). These methods have been applied in synovial fluid and periprosthetic tissue as well as sonicate fluid. The studies, however, are limited, because some positive results on PCR-based testing are difficult to interpret, without otherwise meeting gold standard diagnosis of PJI. This is a particular concern because the methods are at risk of contamination during processing of the specimens. Some studies, however, are reporting increased sensitivity of molecular tests on synovial fluid culture.[43] This has not been reproduced with use of molecular methods on periprosthetic tissue cultures, however.[44,45]

An even newer technique uses metagenomics shotgun sequencing in an effort to identify potentially new and not previously described causes of PJI.[29]

Interleukin 6

Interleukin (IL)-6 is cytokine of recent interest and diagnosis of PJI. Studies have focus on serum and synovial IL-6 levels. Both serum and synovial IL-6 levels seem to have improved diagnostic odds ratios for PJI, and synovial IL-6 seems more specific.[46] Diagnostic values are not yet established for these.

Synovial Fluid Marker Testing

Additional synovial fluid testing has included synovial fluid CRP, with the idea that evaluating the inflammatory state at the joint would give a more specific result than serum biomarkers levels. Synovial fluid CRP seems to perform better than serum CRP based on published diagnostic odds ratio.

A meta-analysis of 13 different synovial fluid test in 33 studies noted high sensitivity for diagnosis of PJI with use of synovial leukocyte count, PMN percentage, CRP, α-defensin, leukocyte esterase, IL-6, and IL-8. In this study, α-defensin showed the highest diagnostic odds ratio for diagnosis of PJI.[47] α-Defensin is of particular interest because it does not seem to fluctuate with the white blood cell count and with combined synovial CRP was useful test in patients with inflammatory conditions.[48] The results similarly do not seem influenced by a previous antimicrobial use either.

TREATMENT

Once a diagnosis of PJI is established, there are several treatment options available. Each case has multiple possible treatment approaches, in terms of both surgical options and antimicrobial use, and choosing the best approach is a combined decision between the patient, the patient's orthopedic surgeon, and an infectious disease specialist, in light of the patient's overall medical condition and goals of care. Although in many cases of infectious diseases the goal is to cure the infection, the best treatment approach to PJI is to have the best functional outcome for the patient with the fewest treatment-related complications. This includes limiting potential morbidity from the treatment approach, and cure of the infection is not always the best approach; instead, the best individual approach may be simply achieving control of infection-related symptoms.

The best surgical approach is decided after reviewing several potential factors. These include the duration of a patient's symptoms, presence of sinus tract, inability to close the soft tissues, the microorganism and its IV and oral antibiotic options, and ability and willingness of a patient to undergo 1 or 2 surgical interventions. These factors, which can influence potential surgical treatment options, are outlined in **Box 1**.

Box 1
Key surgical decision-making factors

Is there available surgical expertise? (can influence decision of OSE vs TSE)

What is the duration of symptoms? (DAIR preferred if short duration of symptoms)

What is the soft tissue coverage? (TSE preferred if concerns present)

Is there a sinus tract present? (TSE preferred)

Is the cause due to a multidrug-resistant organism or lack of oral antibiotic for suppression? (TSE preferred)

What is the patient's ability and willingness to undergo surgery?

Is there any concern regarding stability of the implant? (DAIR considered if no loosening)

Surgical treatment options are generally grouped into 3 approaches.

Débridement, Antibiotic Therapy, Irrigation, and Retention

The first approach involves a combination of DAIR. Patients who benefit from this approach should meet several criteria, including a short duration of symptoms (<3 weeks), absence of sinus tract formation, good soft tissue coverage, stability of the joint, and availability of oral antimicrobial therapy for the identified pathogen.[35] Patients who do not meet these criteria have worse outcomes with this approach, and another approach, like a TSE, described later, should be considered preferential over DAIR. DAIR involves an open arthrotomy, irrigation, and thorough débridement of any infected material and polyethylene liner exchange.

Patients most likely to benefit from this approach are either early PJI cases with less than 3 weeks of symptoms or delayed/late infections occurring after hematogenous seeding of the joint, with short-term symptoms. After surgical intervention, broad-spectrum empiric antimicrobial therapy is transitioned to pathogen-directed antibiotic therapy and is generally administered IV for the first 2 weeks to 6 weeks of therapy.[35] A majority of patients require transition to oral therapy after IV induction course; however, the ideal duration of suppressive therapy is not well defined, although longer courses are typically used for TKA infections. A total of 6 months of combination antibiotic therapy with oral rifampin is recommended for TKA infections versus 3 months of combination with oral rifampin for staphylococcal infections of hip, shoulder, and elbow PJI.[49,50] In cases were highly bioavailable oral antimicrobial therapy is available, particularly with the use of fluoroquinolone/rifampin combination therapy for staphylococcal disease, there are successful reports of avoiding upfront IV antimicrobial therapy altogether.[49] Staphylococcal PJIs treated with DAIR, in patients who are not able to tolerate rifampin as part of their combination therapy, seem to have worse outcomes, and indefinite oral antibiotic suppression for such cases is often used. In addition, microbiology seems to affect the outcome after DAIR, with PJIs due to *Staphylococci*, in particular *S aureus*, vancomycin-resistant *Enterococci*, and fluoroquinolone-resistant gram negative bacilli doing worse compared with other organisms.[50–53] Culture-negative cases also seem to do worse with the DAIR approach, presumable given the difficulty choosing the best antimicrobial regimen.[52] From those that fail DAIR, the next appropriate option is transition to a TSE approach, and TSE surgical approach is utilized in up to 72% of DAIR failures. Salvage options outside repeat TSE include joint resection without reimplantation, arthrodesis, and amputation.[52]

A recently completed randomized trial, awaiting publication, is looking at a completely oral regimen after less than 1 week of IV antibiotic use for management of bone and joint infection, including PJI.[54]

Overall treatment success rate of DAIR has varied widely in the literature over the past few decades, with some inconsistencies in the definition of failure and reports varying from a 34% to a 84% failure rate due to MRSA.[55,56] A recent observational multicenter trial of TKA infection showed a long-term, 4-year expected failure rate of 57.4%.[52]

One-Stage Exchange

OSE is a surgical approach where, during a single operation, an open arthrotomy is performed, followed by complete removal of prosthesis and any previous cement, thorough irrigation, and débridement, followed by implantation of new arthroplasty with antimicrobial loaded cement (chosen with activity against the infective organism). This approach is less frequently used as compared to a TSE in the United States. In general, it is reserved for THA infections, cases of known availability of IV, and oral antimicrobials prior to operation. Antimicrobial treatment courses and duration after OSE also have some variability. Similar to DAIR, an upfront 2-week to 6-week IV antimicrobial is administered, unless there is availability of highly bioavailable oral agents combined with rifampin for staphylococcal infections. Although IDSA guidelines suggest indefinite chronic suppression for these cases, there remains some variability in practice.[35] Treatment success rates of OSE are reported as comparable to those of TSE hip and knee arthroplasty infections, although OSE is more commonly performed for THA infections.[57]

Two-Stage Exchange

The most definitive curative surgical approach for PJI involves a TSE. This approach starts with débridement of infected tissue, removal of old prosthesis, culture collection, removal of old cement, and placement of antibiotic loaded cement spacer into the joint space in an effort to deliver high-dose local antimicrobial therapy and provide structural support. The cement spacer could be either a static spacer or an articulating spacer to provide ongoing mechanical support while the arthroplasty is removed and while delivering local high-level antimicrobial. During this time, in addition to the local antibiotic therapy in the joint, the patient is typically treated with a 4-week to 6-week course of IV antimicrobial therapy. After completion of the IV antimicrobial therapy, the patient is observed off antimicrobial therapy, anywhere from a 2-week to 6-week time period prior to proceeding with the second surgical stage. Observation usually includes clinical evaluation and laboratory work, including inflammatory markers with a goal of identifying those who could benefit from repeat débridement. During the second surgical stage, another opportunity arises at the time of reimplantation surgery to ensure infection is eradicated with intraoperative review of the joint; histopathology is sent, including frozen section, culture collection, and removal of the spacer; and, finally, implantation occurs of new prosthesis if all steps are not concerning for ongoing infection.

TSE is the preferred approach in setting of chronic symptoms of infection, presence of sinus tract, loose prosthesis, and all cases secondary to multidrug-resistant pathogens where antimicrobial options are limited. It is also recommended for cases of fungal PJI.

Success rates with TSE are reported at greater than 85% from several systematic reviews.[58,59] Factors that are associated with TSE failure include presence of sinus tract and prior joint revision history, although many failures actually represent a new infection rather than relapse of the known organism.[60–63]

There is limited evidence that in high-risk patients undergoing TSE, even with negative reimplantation cultures, a short course (varying from 28 days to 3 months) of antimicrobial therapy may decrease the risk of future infection, particularly in those patients with multiple previous revision surgeries and ongoing risk factors.[64,65]

Salvage Surgical Options

In certain cases of PJI, when surgical intervention of any kind is not likely to result in improved level of function, such as in patients who are completely nonambulatory for lower extremity PJI, complete hardware removal without any reimplantation with arthrodesis and even amputation are potential surgical options to consider. These are also the approaches in cases of patients having failed multiple standard TSE who do not have options effective at suppression. When amputation is considered as a treatment option for PJI, seeking a second opinion is generally recommended. Patients undergoing resection arthroplasty and arthrodesis still require 4 weeks to 6 weeks of pathogen-directed therapy. Depending on the level of amputation, if there is persistent proximal intramedullary osteomyelitis, patients may also require treatment of osteomyelitis after surgery.

Nonsurgical Treatment

Although nonsurgical treatment of PJI is not recommended, this approach may be necessary in certain circumstances. For patients who are not believed candidates for surgical intervention, such as in the setting of a palliative approach to their infection and other medical conditions, antimicrobial therapy, as guided by aspiration of the joint and cultures, may be used with appropriate counseling of the patient. These patients are at high risk of relapse of infection and tend to remain on indefinite oral antimicrobial suppression.

SUMMARY

PJI is expected to continue to rise in total numbers managed in the coming years. Diagnosis depends on evaluation of microbiology, inflammatory response, and pathology but diagnostic accuracy is weakened by previous antimicrobial exposure, potential for contamination, and lack of specificity of inflammatory markers. New testing modalities, including molecular methods, promise a quick diagnosis but are limited by potential contamination and lack of susceptibility results. Novel synovial fluid markers show promise as additional armamentarium in the diagnosis of PJI. Surgical and antimicrobial management of each PJI requires personalized evaluation. Good-quality studies aimed at identifying the ideal antimicrobial treatment route and duration for each surgical approach are needed.

REFERENCES

1. Maradit Kremers H, Larson DR, Crowson CS, et al. Prevalence of total hip and knee replacement in the United States. J Bone Joint Surg Am 2015;97(17):1386–97.
2. Kurtz S, Ong K, Lau E, et al. Projections of primary and revision hip and knee arthroplasty in the United States from 2005 to 2030. J Bone Joint Surg Am 2007; 89(4):780–5.
3. Tsaras G, Osmon DR, Mabry T, et al. Incidence, secular trends, and outcomes of prosthetic joint infection: a population-based study, olmsted county, Minnesota, 1969-2007. Infect Control Hosp Epidemiol 2012;33(12):1207–12.
4. Koh CK, Zeng I, Ravi S, et al. Periprosthetic joint infection is the main cause of failure for modern knee arthroplasty: an analysis of 11,134 knees. Clin Orthop Relat Res 2017;475(9):2194–201.
5. Werthel JD, Hatta T, Schoch B, et al. Is previous nonarthroplasty surgery a risk factor for periprosthetic infection in primary shoulder arthroplasty? J Shoulder Elbow Surg 2017;26(4):635–40.

6. Berbari EF, Hanssen AD, Duffy MC, et al. Risk factors for prosthetic joint infection: case-control study. Clin Infect Dis 1998;27(5):1247–54.

7. Jamsen E, Huhtala H, Puolakka T, et al. Risk factors for infection after knee arthroplasty. A register-based analysis of 43,149 cases. J Bone Joint Surg Am 2009; 91(1):38–47.

8. Poss R, Thornhill TS, Ewald FC, et al. Factors influencing the incidence and outcome of infection following total joint arthroplasty. Clin Orthop Relat Res 1984;(182):117–26.

9. Pulido L, Ghanem E, Joshi A, et al. Periprosthetic joint infection: the incidence, timing, and predisposing factors. Clin Orthop Relat Res 2008;466(7):1710–5.

10. Cheng H, Chen BP, Soleas IM, et al. Prolonged operative duration increases risk of surgical site infections: a systematic review. Surg Infect (Larchmt) 2017;18(6): 722–35.

11. Berrios-Torres SI, Umscheid CA, Bratzler DW, et al. Centers for disease control and prevention guideline for the prevention of surgical site infection, 2017. JAMA Surg 2017;152(8):784–91.

12. Mraovic B, Suh D, Jacovides C, et al. Perioperative hyperglycemia and postoperative infection after lower limb arthroplasty. J Diabetes Sci Technol 2011;5(2): 412–8.

13. Kunutsor SK, Whitehouse MR, Blom AW, et al. Patient-related risk factors for periprosthetic joint infection after total joint arthroplasty: a systematic review and meta-analysis. PLoS One 2016;11(3):e0150866.

14. Goodman SM, Springer B, Guyatt G, et al. 2017 American College of Rheumatology/American Association of Hip and Knee Surgeons Guideline for the perioperative management of antirheumatic medication in patients with rheumatic diseases undergoing elective total hip or total knee arthroplasty. J Arthroplasty 2017;32(9):2628–38.

15. Makki D, Elgamal T, Evans P, et al. The orthopaedic manifestation and outcomes of methicillin-sensitive Staphylococcus aureus septicaemia. Bone Joint J 2017; 99-B(11):1545–51.

16. Murdoch DR, Roberts SA, Fowler VG Jr, et al. Infection of orthopedic prostheses after Staphylococcus aureus bacteremia. Clin Infect Dis 2001;32(4):647–9.

17. Stambough JB, Nam D, Warren DK, et al. Decreased hospital costs and surgical site infection incidence with a universal decolonization protocol in primary total joint arthroplasty. J Arthroplasty 2017;32(3):728–34.e1.

18. Mangram AJ, Horan TC, Pearson ML, et al. Guideline for prevention of surgical site infection, 1999. Hospital Infection Control Practices Advisory Committee. Infect Control Hosp Epidemiol 1999;20(4):250–78 [quiz: 279–80].

19. Kurtz SM, Lau E, Watson H, et al. Economic burden of periprosthetic joint infection in the United States. J Arthroplasty 2012;27(8 Suppl):61–5.e1.

20. Parvizi J, Gehrke T. International Consensus Group on Periprosthetic Joint I. Definition of periprosthetic joint infection. J Arthroplasty 2014;29(7):1331.

21. Bedair H, Ting N, Jacovides C, et al. The Mark Coventry Award: diagnosis of early postoperative TKA infection using synovial fluid analysis. Clin Orthop Relat Res 2011;469(1):34–40.

22. Hwang BH, Yoon JY, Nam CH, et al. Fungal peri-prosthetic joint infection after primary total knee replacement. J Bone Joint Surg Br 2012;94(5):656–9.

23. Cobo F, Rodriguez-Granger J, Lopez EM, et al. Candida-induced prosthetic joint infection. A literature review including 72 cases and a case report. Infect Dis (Lond) 2017;49(2):81–94.

24. Azzam K, Parvizi J, Jungkind D, et al. Microbiological, clinical, and surgical features of fungal prosthetic joint infections: a multi-institutional experience. J Bone Joint Surg Am 2009;91(Suppl 6):142–9.

25. Carrega G, Bartolacci V, Burastero G, et al. Prosthetic joint infections due to Mycobacterium tuberculosis: a report of 5 cases. Int J Surg Case Rep 2013; 4(2):178–81.

26. Su JY, Huang TL, Lin SY. Total knee arthroplasty in tuberculous arthritis. Clin Orthop Relat Res 1996;(323):181–7.

27. Chazerain P, Desplaces N, Mamoudy P, et al. Prosthetic total knee infection with a bacillus Calmette Guerin (BCG) strain after BCG therapy for bladder cancer. J Rheumatol 1993;20(12):2171–2.

28. Gomez E, Chiang T, Louie T, et al. Prosthetic Joint Infection due to Mycobacterium bovis after Intravesical Instillation of Bacillus Calmette-Guerin (BCG). Int J Microbiol 2009;2009:527208.

29. Thoendel M, Jeraldo P, Greenwood-Quaintance KE, et al. A novel prosthetic joint infection pathogen, mycoplasma salivarium, identified by metagenomic shotgun sequencing. Clin Infect Dis 2017;65(2):332–5.

30. Berbari EF, Osmon DR, Carr A, et al. Dental procedures as risk factors for prosthetic hip or knee infection: a hospital-based prospective case-control study. Clin Infect Dis 2010;50(1):8–16.

31. Sollecito TP, Abt E, Lockhart PB, et al. The use of prophylactic antibiotics prior to dental procedures in patients with prosthetic joints: Evidence-based clinical practice guideline for dental practitioners–a report of the American Dental Association Council on Scientific Affairs. J Am Dent Assoc 2015;146(1):11–6.e18.

32. Wilson W, Taubert KA, Gewitz M, et al. Prevention of infective endocarditis: guidelines from the American Heart Association: a guideline from the American Heart Association Rheumatic Fever, Endocarditis, and Kawasaki Disease Committee, Council on Cardiovascular Disease in the Young, and the Council on Clinical Cardiology, Council on Cardiovascular Surgery and Anesthesia, and the Quality of Care and Outcomes Research Interdisciplinary Working Group. Circulation 2007;116(15):1736–54.

33. Watters W 3rd, Rethman MP, Hanson NB, et al. Prevention of orthopaedic implant infection in patients undergoing dental procedures. J Am Acad Orthop Surg 2013;21(3):180–9.

34. Cordero-Ampuero J, Gonzalez-Fernandez E, Martinez-Velez D, et al. Are antibiotics necessary in hip arthroplasty with asymptomatic bacteriuria? Seeding risk with/without treatment. Clin Orthop Relat Res 2013;471(12):3822–9.

35. Osmon DR, Berbari EF, Berendt AR, et al. Diagnosis and management of prosthetic joint infection: clinical practice guidelines by the Infectious Diseases Society of America. Clin Infect Dis 2013;56(1):e1–25.

36. Parvizi J, Zmistowski B, Berbari EF, et al. New definition for periprosthetic joint infection: from the Workgroup of the Musculoskeletal Infection Society. Clin Orthop Relat Res 2011;469(11):2992–4.

37. Malekzadeh D, Osmon DR, Lahr BD, et al. Prior use of antimicrobial therapy is a risk factor for culture-negative prosthetic joint infection. Clin Orthop Relat Res 2010;468(8):2039–45.

38. Schinsky MF, Della Valle CJ, Sporer SM, et al. Perioperative testing for joint infection in patients undergoing revision total hip arthroplasty. J Bone Joint Surg Am 2008;90(9):1869–75.

39. Ghanem E, Parvizi J, Burnett RS, et al. Cell count and differential of aspirated fluid in the diagnosis of infection at the site of total knee arthroplasty. J Bone Joint Surg Am 2008;90(8):1637–43.

40. Tsaras G, Maduka-Ezeh A, Inwards CY, et al. Utility of intraoperative frozen section histopathology in the diagnosis of periprosthetic joint infection: a systematic review and meta-analysis. J Bone Joint Surg Am 2012;94(18):1700–11.

41. Feldman DS, Lonner JH, Desai P, et al. The role of intraoperative frozen sections in revision total joint arthroplasty. J Bone Joint Surg Am 1995;77(12):1807–13.

42. Hughes HC, Newnham R, Athanasou N, et al. Microbiological diagnosis of prosthetic joint infections: a prospective evaluation of four bacterial culture media in the routine laboratory. Clin Microbiol Infect 2011;17(10):1528–30.

43. Greenwood-Quaintance KE, Uhl JR, Hanssen AD, et al. Diagnosis of prosthetic joint infection by use of PCR-electrospray ionization mass spectrometry. J Clin Microbiol 2014;52(2):642–9.

44. Ryu SY, Greenwood-Quaintance KE, Hanssen AD, et al. Low sensitivity of periprosthetic tissue PCR for prosthetic knee infection diagnosis. Diagn Microbiol Infect Dis 2014;79(4):448–53.

45. Bemer P, Plouzeau C, Tande D, et al. Evaluation of 16S rRNA gene PCR sensitivity and specificity for diagnosis of prosthetic joint infection: a prospective multicenter cross-sectional study. J Clin Microbiol 2014;52(10):3583–9.

46. Randau TM, Friedrich MJ, Wimmer MD, et al. Interleukin-6 in serum and in synovial fluid enhances the differentiation between periprosthetic joint infection and aseptic loosening. PLoS One 2014;9(2):e89045.

47. Lee YS, Koo KH, Kim HJ, et al. Synovial fluid biomarkers for the diagnosis of periprosthetic joint infection: a systematic review and meta-analysis. J Bone Joint Surg Am 2017;99(24):2077–84.

48. Deirmengian C, Kardos K, Kilmartin P, et al. Combined measurement of synovial fluid alpha-Defensin and C-reactive protein levels: highly accurate for diagnosing periprosthetic joint infection. J Bone Joint Surg Am 2014;96(17):1439–45.

49. Lora-Tamayo J, Euba G, Cobo J, et al. Short- versus long-duration levofloxacin plus rifampicin for acute staphylococcal prosthetic joint infection managed with implant retention: a randomised clinical trial. Int J Antimicrob Agents 2016; 48(3):310–6.

50. Chaussade H, Uckay I, Vuagnat A, et al. Antibiotic therapy duration for prosthetic joint infections treated by debridement and implant retention (DAIR): Similar long-term remission for 6 weeks as compared to 12 weeks. Int J Infect Dis 2017;63: 37–42.

51. Jaen N, Martinez-Pastor JC, Munoz-Mahamud E, et al. Long-term outcome of acute prosthetic joint infections due to gram-negative bacilli treated with retention of prosthesis. Rev Esp Quimioter 2012;25(3):194–8.

52. Urish KL, Bullock AG, Kreger AM, et al. A multicenter study of irrigation and debridement in total knee arthroplasty periprosthetic joint infection: treatment failure is high. J Arthroplasty 2018;33(4):1154–9.

53. Soriano A, Garcia S, Bori G, et al. Treatment of acute post-surgical infection of joint arthroplasty. Clin Microbiol Infect 2006;12(9):930–3.

54. Li HK, Scarborough M, Zambellas R, et al. Oral versus intravenous antibiotic treatment for bone and joint infections (OVIVA): study protocol for a randomised controlled trial. Trials 2015;16:583.

55. Kuiper JW, Vos SJ, Saouti R, et al. Prosthetic joint-associated infections treated with DAIR (debridement, antibiotics, irrigation, and retention): analysis of risk factors and local antibiotic carriers in 91 patients. Acta Orthop 2013;84(4):380–6.

56. Bradbury T, Fehring TK, Taunton M, et al. The fate of acute methicillin-resistant Staphylococcus aureus periprosthetic knee infections treated by open debridement and retention of components. J Arthroplasty 2009;24(6 Suppl):101–4.
57. Nagra NS, Hamilton TW, Ganatra S, et al. One-stage versus two-stage exchange arthroplasty for infected total knee arthroplasty: a systematic review. Knee Surg Sports Traumatol Arthrosc 2016;24(10):3106–14.
58. Lange J, Troelsen A, Thomsen RW, et al. Chronic infections in hip arthroplasties: comparing risk of reinfection following one-stage and two-stage revision: a systematic review and meta-analysis. Clin Epidemiol 2012;4:57–73.
59. Jamsen E, Stogiannidis I, Malmivaara A, et al. Outcome of prosthesis exchange for infected knee arthroplasty: the effect of treatment approach. Acta Orthop 2009;80(1):67–77.
60. Betsch BY, Eggli S, Siebenrock KA, et al. Treatment of joint prosthesis infection in accordance with current recommendations improves outcome. Clin Infect Dis 2008;46(8):1221–6.
61. Mortazavi SM, Vegari D, Ho A, et al. Two-stage exchange arthroplasty for infected total knee arthroplasty: predictors of failure. Clin Orthop Relat Res 2011;469(11): 3049–54.
62. Hirakawa K, Stulberg BN, Wilde AH, et al. Results of 2-stage reimplantation for infected total knee arthroplasty. J Arthroplasty 1998;13(1):22–8.
63. Bejon P, Berendt A, Atkins BL, et al. Two-stage revision for prosthetic joint infection: predictors of outcome and the role of reimplantation microbiology. J Antimicrob Chemother 2010;65(3):569–75.
64. Frank JM, Kayupov E, Moric M, et al. The Mark Coventry, MD, award: oral antibiotics reduce reinfection after two-stage exchange: a multicenter, randomized controlled trial. Clin Orthop Relat Res 2017;475(1):56–61.
65. Zywiel MG, Johnson AJ, Stroh DA, et al. Prophylactic oral antibiotics reduce reinfection rates following two-stage revision total knee arthroplasty. Int Orthop 2011; 35(1):37–42.

Neurosurgical Device-Related Infections

Jessica Seidelman, MD[a,b,*], Sarah S. Lewis, MD, MPH[a,b]

KEYWORDS

- Infection • Meningitis • Ventriculitis • Cerebrospinal fluid shunt
- External ventriculostomy drain • Lumbar drain • Deep brain stimulator

KEY POINTS

- The increasing use of central nervous system devices is associated with an increasing incidence of device-related infections.
- Causative pathogens are related to the timing of surgery and route of infection.
- Patients with central nervous system device infections may not present with classic signs or symptoms of meningitis, which makes diagnosis challenging.
- Periprocedural antibiotics and adherence to perioperative control measures decrease the risk of central nervous system device infections.

INTRODUCTION

Neurosurgical devices play an important role in the diagnosis and treatment of many neurologic conditions. The evolution of these devices has led to improvements that maximize their clinical benefits and minimize adverse effects and has made them increasingly popular. However, the introduction of any nonbiologic material into the human body creates an opportunity for infection. Unfortunately, infection from neurosurgical devices is associated with increased morbidity and mortality.[1] Therefore, understanding the presentation, diagnosis, and treatment of the increasing number of patients with neurologic device infections is critical.

In this review article, we discuss the epidemiology, microbiology, diagnosis, treatment and prevention of infections associated with cerebrospinal fluid (CSF) shunts, CSF drains, and deep brain stimulators (DBS).

The authors have no conflicts of interest or financial support to disclose.

[a] Division of Infectious Diseases, Department of Medicine, Duke University School of Medicine, Duke University Medical Center, PO Box 102359, Durham, NC 27710, USA; [b] Division of Infectious Diseases, Duke Center for Antimicrobial Stewardship and Infection Prevention, Duke University Medical Center, PO Box 102359, Durham, NC 27710, USA
* Corresponding author. Department of Medicine, Division of Infectious Diseases, Duke University Medical Center, PO Box 102359, Durham, NC 27710.
E-mail address: jessica.seidelman@duke.edu

Infect Dis Clin N Am 32 (2018) 861–876
https://doi.org/10.1016/j.idc.2018.06.006
0891-5520/18/© 2018 Elsevier Inc. All rights reserved.

SHUNTS

CSF shunts are most commonly placed for the treatment of hydrocephalus.[2] However, they are also used to relieve increased intracranial pressure in the setting of tumors, subarachnoid hemorrhage, head injuries, and intraventricular hemorrhage.[3] All CSF shunts have 2 major components: proximal end and distal end. The proximal end common enters the lateral ventricle via a burr hole. The connected distal portion can terminate in the peritoneum (ventriculoperitoneal shunt), pleura (ventriculopleural shunt), or right atrium (ventriculoatrial shunt). The entire shunt is internalized, but can be accessed with a needle via a subcutaneous ventricular reservoir.[3]

Epidemiology

The first CSF shunt surgeries were performed in the 1950s and were commonly complicated by infection. Since that time, there have been many advances in neurosurgical techniques and shunt design, but infection remains a major complication. The incidence of shunt-related infections is as high as 4% to 17%.[4]

Risk factors for developing shunt infections are generally categorized as host specific or procedure specific. Host-related risk factors include premature birth, especially when associated with intraventricular hemorrhage, younger age, previous shunt infection, and etiology of hydrocephalus, including purulent meningitis, hemorrhage, and myelomeningocele.[5–7] Procedure-related risk factors include a shunt revision procedure, especially those undergoing 3 or more revisions; duration of operation; use of neuroendoscope; experience of neurosurgeon; and insertion of catheter below the T7 vertebral body in a ventriculoatrial shunt.[6–8]

Microbiology

Shunt-related infections occur by 3 major routes: (1) introduction of infection at the time of surgery, (2) hematogenous spread from a distant site, or (3) contiguous spread from a nearby source. The most common infecting pathogens vary based on the mode of infection. Infections occurring at the time of shunt placement typically present within 1 month after surgery,[9,10] and are most commonly caused by skin flora including coagulase-negative staphylococci, *Staphylococcus aureus*, and *Propionibacterium acnes*.[11–13] The incidence of shunt infections owing to gram-negative rods is lower at 6% to 20%.[14]

Hematogenous spread from a distal focus of infection is of particular concern with ventriculoatrial shunts. These infections can occur any time after shunt implantation, even years after the surgery. The microorganisms involved depend on the secondary site of infection. For example, ventriculoatrial shunt infections caused by *Haemophilus influenza* and *Streptococcus pneumoniae* have been reported after acute otitis media.[15]

Last, shunts can become colonized from a nearby source of infection via contiguous spread. Bowel perforation or peritonitis can seed the distal end of ventriculoperitoneal shunts and cause polymicrobial infections, including gram-negative organisms. The proximal portion of CSF shunts can be seeded from scalp wounds, by accessing the ventricular reservoir, or after ENT surgery.[15–17] As with infections from hematogenous spread, these infections can occur at any time after shunt placement and the suspected bacterial pathogens depend on the primary infection's etiology.

Diagnosis

Clinical diagnosis

CSF shunt infections need to be diagnosed quickly and accurately to make appropriate medical and surgical treatment plans. However, diagnosis can be challenging because signs, symptoms, and laboratory findings commonly associated with meningitis are not always present.

Patients with CSF shunt infections may present with few or no symptoms.[14] Conen and colleagues[14] found that neck stiffness (45%), decrease in Glasgow Coma Scale (31%), headache (21%), or nausea (14%) were not reliably present in patients with shunt-related CSF infections. Furthermore, this same study found that 36% of patient had no neurologic signs or symptoms at the time of initial presentation. The lack of meningeal or systemic symptoms may be related to the altered or absent connection between ventricles and meninges as well as the low virulence of the organisms that are commonly associated with CSF shunt infections (eg, coagulase-negative staphylococci and P acnes).[18] Therefore, health care providers should not exclude the possibility of a CSF shunt infection owing to the lack of traditional meningitic signs/symptoms.

Although many of the classic meningeal signs or symptoms may be absent with CSF shunt infections, there are some clinical clues that, if present, should raise suspicion for a CSF shunt infection. Two recent independent studies reported that fever was the most common sign of CSF shunt infection, present in 78% and 89% of patients.[10,14] Moreover, the magnitude of fever is important. A temperature of greater than 39.4°C accurately distinguished bacterial from chemical meningitis in patients with CSF shunts.[19]

Local signs of infection surrounding the proximal portion or distal portion of the shunt, if present, increase the suspicion for shunt-related infection. Conen and colleagues[14] found that erythema, local pain, swelling, and/or purulent drainage involving the proximal shunt implantation site were present in 49% of patients with confirmed CSF shunt infections. Likewise, patients with ventriculoperitoneal or ventriculopleural shunts may present with signs of peritonitis or pleuritis, respectively.[4] Specifically, patients with ventriculoperitoneal shunts may present with abdominal pain and patients with ventriculopleural shunts may report chest pain that is worst with inspiration.

In summary, shunt infections can cause few or no symptoms. Clinically, no individual sign or symptom has both high sensitivity and high specificity for the diagnosis of CSF shunt infections. As such, providers should have a low threshold to perform additional diagnostic testing in patients with CSF shunts who present with new symptoms that are not otherwise explained.

Laboratory studies

CSF cultures from the shunt are critical in establishing the diagnosis of shunt infections. Cultures can be positive even in the absence of CSF pleocytosis or CSF chemistry aberrancies.[4] CSF cultures should be kept for at least 10 days because a lack of initial growth can be due to slow-growing organisms such as P acnes or as a result of antibiotic administration before CSF culture collection.[4] One study found that CSF cultures obtained before antibiotic therapy had a sensitivity of 88%. This decreased to 70% if cultures were obtained after the administration of antibiotics.[20]

Nucleic acid amplification tests (NAATs) performed on CSF may be helpful in the diagnosis of bacterial meningitis in patients with neurologic devices, particularly when standard CSF cultures are negative. Investigators performed both 16sRNA polymerase chain reaction and standard cultures on CSF of patients with suspected infections of either an external ventricular drain (EVD) or ventriculoperitoneal shunt and found that 49% of patient samples had a negative culture but a positive polymerase chain reaction result.[21] Because NAAT tests do not provide drug susceptibility information, NAAT testing does not replace CSF culture. However, NAAT testing may be pursued when standard CSF cultures are negative and suspicion for CSF shunt infection remains high.

CSF white blood cell count is an unreliable means of diagnosing CSF shunt infections. Patients with recent device placement may exhibit CSF pleocytosis, which can be caused by inflammation from infection or inflammation from recent catheter placement. Although Forgacs and colleagues[19] found that a CSF white blood cell count of greater than 7500/μL was only found in patients with bacterial ventriculitis (vs chemical meningitis), Conen and colleagues[14] found no significant pleocytosis in 20% of patients with confirmed CSF shunt-associated infections. Therefore, the absence of CSF pleocytosis does not exclude a CSF shunt infection.

CSF lactate and serum procalcitonin levels are tests that clinicians have investigated to help delineate the presence of a CSF shunt infection. However, current studies have shown mixed results. Additional research is needed before these 2 tests can reliably be used to diagnose CSF shunt infections.

Radiology

Neuroimaging studies are rarely definitive in the diagnosis of CSF shunt infections. However, they are often obtained and can support the diagnosis. Specifically, plain radiographs or computed tomography scans may show evidence of retained hardware that could be serving as a nidus of infection. Neuroimaging may also show contiguous spread of infection from another area. Patients with ventriculoperitoneal shunts presenting with abdominal pain should also have an ultrasound or computed tomography scan of the abdomen to look for loculations adjacent to the terminus of the catheter because this symptom may be an indication of infection.[22] Finally, imaging may show complications such as hydrocephalus that sometimes occur in the setting of shunt infections or malfunctions.[23] Therefore, although neuroimaging studies are infrequently definitive, they can provide useful information if certain findings are present.

Treatment

There are currently no randomized trials that address the optimal management of CSF shunt infections. Treatment of CSF shunt infections include antibiotics in addition to the removal and replacement of the infected hardware.[24,25]

Antibiotics

If a CSF shunt infection is suspected, empiric antibiotics should be administered after appropriate cultures are obtained even before confirmation of the diagnosis, because a delay in therapy can result in significant morbidity and mortality. Current Infectious Diseases Society of America guidelines recommend empiric treatment with intravenous vancomycin with a goal trough of 15 to 20 mg/dL and a concurrent gram-negative antibiotic based on local antimicrobial susceptibility patterns.[4] Examples of appropriate gram-negative antibiotics to cover health care–associated gram-negative bacilli are ceftazidime, cefepime, or meropenem. Aztreonam or ciprofloxacin are appropriate alternatives for adults with a severe beta-lactam allergy.[4]

Antibiotic therapy should be tailored based on culture results and specific agents should be selected based on CSF penetration and patient allergy profile, consistent with the current Infectious Diseases Society of America guideline recommendations.[4] In the event that CSF cultures remain negative and there remains a strong suspicion of a CNS infection, empiric vancomycin therapy should be continued for presumed staphylococcal infection in addition to a gram-negative antibiotic based on local susceptibility data.[4] Intraventricular administration of antibiotics is not currently approved by the US Food and Drug Administration and there is insufficient evidence to recommend their routine use except when the infection responds poorly to systemic antibiotic treatment alone. However, intraventricular therapy has been used in some difficult-to-treat cases.[26,27]

There are no randomized trials that have been used to determine the optimal duration of antibiotic therapy.[4,25] However, a prospective observational study on patients with shunt infections found that the reinfection rates for antibiotic duration of 10 days or less, 11 to 20 days, and 21 days or more were 28.5%, 23.3%, and 27.7%, respectively.[2] Currently, the 2017 Infectious Diseases Society of America guidelines recommend the durations of therapy according to CSF findings and causative organism provided in **Table 1**.[4]

Patients with shunt infections should be monitored clinically to look for ongoing indications of infection. Clinicians should obtain repeat CSF cultures every 48 to 72 hours to document clearance.[4]

Surgical management

Management of shunt infections without catheter removal has been attempted periodically throughout the years. This approach avoids the morbidity of additional operations. However, success rates without device removal are low and lead to poor outcomes. The low cure rates are likely because many of the typical causative pathogens form biofilms and cannot be cleared from the catheter with antibiotics alone. As such, removal of infected devices has become a critical element in the treatment of shunt infections.[24,28] Typically, a 2-stage shunt replacement is performed in which the shunt is removed and an EVD placed temporarily until a new shunt is placed. A 1-stage shunt replacement is when the infected shunt is replaced with a new shunt during the same operation. A retrospective study of 50 patients by James and colleagues[29] found that patients treated with shunt removal and antibiotics versus patients treated with antibiotics alone had treatment response rates of 95% and 35%, respectively. A more recent retrospective study by Pelegrin and colleagues[26] evaluated the risk factors that predicted treatment failure in ventriculoperitoneal shunt

Table 1
Infectious Diseases Society of America CSF shunt infection treatment duration recommendations

Causative Organism(s)	CSF Findings and Systemic Symptoms	Duration of Therapy[b]
Coagulase negative staphylococci or *Propionibacterium acnes*	No or minimal CSF pleocytosis Normal CSF glucose Few clinical symptoms	10 d
Coagulase-negative staphylococci or *P acnes*	Significant CSF pleocytosis Low CSF glucose Significant clinical symptoms	10–14 d
Staphylococcus aureus or gram-negative bacilli	Without or without significant CSF pleocytosis Low CSF glucose Clinical symptoms	10–14 d[a]

Abbreviation: CSF, cerebrospinal fluid.
[a] Some experts believe that gram-negative bacilli central nervous system infections should be treated for 21 days.
[b] Patients with persistently positive CSF cultures, antibiotics therapy should extend to 10 to 14 days from the date of the last positive culture. Patients who have a delayed or incomplete response to therapy may benefit from longer courses of antibiotics.
Data from Tunkel AR, Hasbun R, Bhimraj A, et al. 2017 Infectious diseases society of America's clinical practice guidelines for healthcare-associated ventriculitis and meningitis. Clin Infect Dis 2017;64(6):e34-65.

infections. The only risk factor associated with treatment failure in this analysis was shunt retention. Moreover, failure occurred in 68% of patients with a 1-stage shunt replacement compared with 11% of patients who had a 2-stage shunt exchange. Given the higher cure rates, shunt removal is the standard of care in the treatment of shunt infections.

There are no randomized trials that have defined the optimal timing of a new shunt placement, and this is typically determined based on the initial severity of infection, pathogen, and response to treatment (**Table 2**).[4] Patients should be closely monitored after placement of the new shunt to ensure that there are no recurrent signs of infection.

CEREBROSPINAL FLUID DRAINS

CSF drains are critical medical devices used for therapeutic diversion of CSF to prevent damage from high CSF pressure, as monitoring devices for CSF pressure, and to directly access CSF for medication administration. Although CSF drains are necessary and often used to prevent or minimize brain damage and save lives, they increase the risk of infection.

CSF drains typically consist of 2 components: a proximal end and a distal end. The proximal end is typically placed into either the cerebral ventricle (EVD) or the lumbar subarachnoid space (lumbar drain [LD]).[30] The distal end of the catheter is tunneled a distance subcutaneously before exiting the skin and connected to an external collection system. In addition to a collection bag for CSF, the external component has ports to measure CSF pressure, sample CSF, and inject medication into the CSF.

Epidemiology

Incidence rates for EVD-related meningitis are reported to range from 2% to 22% versus 4% to 7% for LD-associated infections.[31] The large range of reported incidence rates is likely due the various definitions of infection among studies. The lower incidence of LD-associated infections is attributed to the lower risk patient group that

Table 2
Infectious Diseases Society of America guideline recommendations for timing of new shunt placement

Pathogen	CSF Findings	Repeat CSF Culture	When New Shunt Can Be Placed
Coagulase-negative staphylococci or *Propionibacterium acnes*	No CSF abnormalities	Negative at 48 h	Day 3 after removal of infected shunt
Coagulase-negative staphylococci or *P acnes*	CSF abnormalities	Negative	After 7 d of antibiotics
Coagulase-negative staphylococci or *P acnes*	CSF abnormalities	Positive	Antibiotics for 7–10 d after repeat cultures are negative
Staphylococcus aureus	With or without CSF abnormalities	Negative	10 d after CSF cultures are negative
Gram-negative bacilli	With or without CSF abnormalities	Negative	10 d after CSF cultures are negative

Abbreviation: CSF, cerebrospinal fluid.
Data from Tunkel AR, Hasbun R, Bhimraj A, et al. 2017 Infectious diseases society of America's clinical practice guidelines for healthcare-associated ventriculitis and meningitis. Clin Infect Dis 2017;64(6):e34-65.

undergo LD placement (ie, for diagnosis of normal pressure hydrocephalus) compared with the group of patients undergoing EVD placement.

There are several factors associated with an increased risk of CSF drain–related infections. These issues relate to the indication for catheter placement, the frequency of drain manipulation or sampling, and the duration of catheterization. CSF drain placement for the treatment of intraventricular hemorrhage and subarachnoid hemorrhage carry a higher risk of subsequent infection compared with other indications for CSF drain placement.[32] Other risk factors for infection are CSF leakage from the ventriculostomy site, CSF catheter irrigation, frequent CSF sampling, and the severity of underling the illness, including systemic infections.[4,30,33,34] Specific to patients with LDs, the risk of infection increases when the external drainage system is disconnected from the catheter.[35] Although there is some ongoing debate as to whether a longer duration of drain placement is truly a risk factor for CSF drain infections, most studies consider catheter presence of longer than 5 days to be a risk factor for infection.[4,30,36] Health care providers should have a higher suspicion for CSF drain infections when patients present with 1 or more of these risk factors.

Microbiology

As with CSF shunt infections, CSF drain infections are typically caused by microorganisms introduced through the skin at the time of drain placement. Microorganisms may also enter the catheter through retrograde contamination from a nearby source of infection or during routine care/manipulation of the external drain system.

Inoculation of the CSF drain with bacteria at the time of surgical placement is the most common cause of CSF drain infections. Unlike CSF shunt infections, there is no clear delineation of what constitutes an early infection because the majority of CSF drains only remain in place for days to weeks. About one-half of CSF drain infections are caused by coagulase-negative staphylococci and about one-third are caused by S aureus.[37,38] Diphtheroids may also be pathogenic in CSF drain infections.[4]

Retrograde infection of the drain catheter can occur if there is skin breakdown adjacent to the site of drain placement or if bacteria is introduced through the catheter during manipulation or routine care. As with perioperative contamination, gram-positive organisms also cause the majority of retrograde infections.[4] Although the majority of CSF drain infections are caused by gram-positive organisms, the rate of CSF drain infections caused by gram-negative organisms is increasing. Gram-negative bacilli (namely Escherichia coli and Klebsiella spp) are responsible for 6% to 20% of CSF drain infections.[10,39] A prospective study by Lyke and colleagues[33] found that the majority of their hospital's EVD infections (9 of 11 cases) were due to gram-negative organisms. They hypothesized that this may be because antibiotic prophylaxis before catheter placement is mainly directed against gram-positive organisms. Another potential explanation from their study was the prolonged hospitalization duration, which may have led to gram-negative microbial colonization of the patients and their drains.

Diagnosis

Clinical diagnosis

As with shunt-related infections, the clinical signs and symptoms of CSF drain infections are nonspecific and often overlap with the neurologic conditions for which patients require the CSF drains. In retrospective study of EVD infections by Walti and colleagues,[40] a decrease in the Glasgow Coma Scale score and other neurologic signs were present in fewer than one-third of patients diagnosed with EVD infection.

However, researchers found that fever was present in 79% of patients with an EVD infection versus only 15% of patients with EVDs in place and no evidence of infection. A cohort study by Schade and colleagues[41] also found that fever was present in every patient with a CSF drain infection. However, other studies have found that there is not a single clinical parameter that can reliably predict or exclude CSF drain infections.[42,43] Because there is no clinical parameter that can consistently diagnose CSF drain infections, clinicians must rely on other methods of diagnosis.

Culture and gram stain Definitive CSF drain infections are defined as a positive CSF culture obtained from the CSF drain with associated CSF pleocytosis.[30,34] A positive gram stain or culture is highly specific but poorly sensitive for CSF drain-associated infections.[44,45] Therefore, a positive gram stain or culture can be very useful, but a negative result does not rule out infection.

NAAT is another diagnostic test that shows promise in diagnosing bacterial CSF drain infections. Deutch and colleagues[46] looked at patients with suspected CSF drain infections and tested CSF samples using traditional CSF culture and polymerase chain reaction. The authors concluded that polymerase chain reaction increased the yield of causative pathogens when used in conjunction with CSF culture. Polymerase chain reaction was particularly useful in identifying fastidious gram-negative bacteria. As with CSF shunt infections, NAAT may be useful when standard cultures are negative. However, this test is not available commercially for CSF samples and additional studies are needed to better assess its usefulness.

Most authors suggest performing a complete CSF diagnostic workup if a CSF drain-associated infection is suspected, including leukocyte count and differential, glucose, protein, and gram stain/culture.[47,48] CSF parameters in CSF drain infections vary greatly and none have been shown to be predictive of infection.[42,45] Schade and colleagues[48] took daily CSF samples from patients with external CSF drains and prospectively looked for microbiologic evidence of device infection. CSF was analyzed for leukocyte count, protein concentration, glucose concentration, and ratio of CSF glucose to serum glucose. The authors found no differences between the CSF profiles of patients with culture-proven infection and those without culture-proven infection from 3 days preceding infection diagnosis through 3 days after diagnosis of infection. Pfisterer and colleagues[47] also found a lack of CSF differences between patients with EVD infection and those without evidence of EVD infection; however, they did find that CSF cell count was significantly correlated with the occurrence of a positive CSF culture. Pfausler and colleagues[44] investigated the usefulness of the ratio of CSF leukocytes to erythrocytes as a means to diagnose CSF drain infection. However, the ratio of cells did not predict infection at any of the time points studied. Currently, there does not seem to be evidence that supports the use of specific CSF parameters to diagnose or exclude an EVD-associated infection.

The serum procalcitonin level is another diagnostic metric that has been suggested to aid in the diagnosis of CSF drain infections. Omar and colleagues[49] studied patients with severe head trauma and subsequent CSF drain placement. Researchers found that patients with negative CSF cultures had a mean serum procalcitonin level of less than 2.0 ng/mL, compared with patients with positive cultures had a mean serum procalcitonin level of 4.18 ng/mL. Berger and colleagues[50] also found that serum procalcitonin levels were significantly higher (4.7 vs 0.2 ng/mL) in patients with proven bacterial CSF drain infections compared with those without culture-proven infections. However, Martinez and colleagues[51] did not find that serum procalcitonin alone was a helpful in diagnosing CSF drain infections. Unfortunately, more data are needed before procalcitonin can be reliably used alone by clinicians to diagnose CSF drain infections.

Routine surveillance of CSF fluid parameters in patients with CSF drains without signs of infection is not recommended.[4] Results from surveillance samples do not reliably predict infection and can increase the chance of iatrogenic infection. A prospective study found that daily routine CSF analysis for prediction or diagnosis of CSF drain-associated infection was not clinically helpful.[48] This same study reported no differences in daily CSF chemistries between patients with and without CSF drain infections.

Treatment

Antibiotics

Overall, the recommendations for empiric and targeted systemic antibiotics are the same for CSF drain infections and shunt infections, as discussed elsewhere in this article. As with CSF shunt infections, the use of intraventricular antibiotics is recommended by the most recent Infectious Diseases Society of America guidelines for CSF drain-associated infections that respond poorly to systemic antibiotics alone.[4] Intraventricular antibiotics for patients with EVD ventriculitis are also endorsed by the Neurosurgery Working Party of the British Society for Antimicrobial Chemotherapy.[52] Studies advocate that intraventricular antibiotics are not associated with severe or irreversible toxicity.[53] There is also some research that shows better pharmacodynamics and similar efficacy of intraventricular antibiotics compared with intravenous antibiotics.[44,54] However, as discussed elsewhere in this article, intraventricular antibiotics are not currently approved by the US Food and Drug Administration and are not used routinely to treat CSF drain infections.

Surgical management

Occasionally, antibiotics alone are not sufficient to treat CSF drain infections and device removal should be considered.[55] Beer and colleagues[56] recommend considering CSF drain removal when CSF is purulent and if patients have an inadequate response to antimicrobial therapy.

Implanted Electrodes

DBS was introduced in 1987 for the treatment of Parkinson's disease. Today, patients receive DBS for treatment of other conditions including movement disorders and chronic pain.[57] However, as with all implanted devices, infection is a known complication.

Each DBS consists of 3 essential parts: an intracranial lead, a connector, and an implanted pulse generator. The pulse generator is typically implanted in the infraclavicular region, similar to a pacemaker device. Infection can involve all 3 elements of the DBS, but infection of the pulse generator is the most common.[4]

Epidemiology

Incidence data for DBS-related infections is difficult to interpret owing to the lack of a standardized definition. Some groups report superficial skin infections at incision sites, whereas others only report infections involving the hardware.[36] That being said, reported incidence proportions range from 0.62% to 14.3%.[36] The wide variation in incidence likely also reflects the multitude of surgical techniques, varying antimicrobial prophylaxis practices, and lack of a standard definition.

To date, the medical literature has not identified any definitive risk factors for DBS infections. The dearth of conclusive evidence is attributed to the lack of a universal reporting system for DBS infections and the small numbers of patients in individual studies.

Microbiology

The majority of DBS infections are the result of skin pathogens. *S aureus, S epidermidis,* and *P acnes* are the most common organisms associated with these infections.[57–59] However, gram-negative organisms and mycobacteria have been isolated as well.[60,61]

Diagnosis

Clinical diagnosis Infections are commonly found at 1 of 3 sites: the pulse generator, the connector site, or on the scalp overlying the site where the lead exits the brain. Infections can also be categorized as early or late. Early infections occur within 30 days to 6 months of implantation, whereas late infections occur more than 6 months after device placement.

Early infections typically present with erythema, edema, and/or drainage from the intracranial lead or implanted generator. Wound dehiscence or exposure of hardware are other possible indications of infection. Rarely, patients can present with focal neurologic symptoms or seizures caused by an intracranial abscess.[36] In contrast, late infections occur more than 6 months after implantation and are often but not always preceded by manipulation of the device. For example, battery exchanges can lead to infections years after implantation. Erosion of the skin surrounding any of the 3 components is the most common presentation of late infection.[57] These patients commonly present with nonhealing wounds overlying a device component.

Laboratory studies As with many other surgical site infections, surgical cultures are the most reliable diagnostic tests. Surgical cultures can also provide microorganism sensitivity information to determine final antimicrobial therapy.

Imaging Brain imaging is indicated when clinical presentation is indicative of an intracranial infection, specifically a brain abscess. MRI is more sensitive than computed tomography scanning for the diagnosis of a brain abscess. Despite initial concerns that MRI is not a safe modality to use in patients with DBS, studies have shown that this procedure is well-tolerated by this patient population.[62,63]

Treatment

Infections of DBS hardware can lead to significant morbidity from system removal and resultant poor control of the underlying illness, prolonged hospitalization, prolonged antimicrobial use, and repeated surgical procedures. As with other device-related infections, the 2 main components of treatment are antimicrobials and device removal.

Antibiotic therapy consists of empiric and subsequent targeted treatment. Empiric therapy should cover the most common organisms associated with DBS-associated infections, specifically staphylococci and *P acnes.*[57] Once susceptibility data are available, health care providers should switch antibiotics to target recovered microorganisms.

The duration of antibiotic therapy ranges from 2 to 4 weeks after removal of infected hardware.[4,57] Two weeks is generally reserved for infection that is limited to the pulse generator pocket without any evidence of infection involving the connector or intracranial lead. Six weeks of antibiotics is required if there is evidence of intracranial infection or cranial osteomyelitis.

The central issue of management revolves around the need to remove infected implants, the timing of removal, and the extent of the removal (partial or complete system removal). The decision to remove a device is not insignificant owing to the need for repeated neurosurgical interventions, the cost of the devices, and the burden placed on the patient. The extent to which device removal is necessary depends on whether the intracranial lead is infected. For infection that only involves the generator site, patients should have a trial of brain lead–sparing surgery with removal of only the battery and extension. However, if the surgeon finds gross evidence of infection at the connector site or around the burr hole, the entire system should be removed. Without complete device removal, these patients are likely to develop recurrent infection.[36] The main distinction in these settings is that the intracranial lead is infected.

There are no randomized controlled trials that discuss the appropriate time to reimplant a DBS after infection. Expert opinion suggests that reimplantation is appropriate 3 to 6 months after the completion of antibacterial treatment.[4,57]

Prevention

Although the risk of infection exists with neurologic devices, there are opportunities to decrease this risk with appropriate antibiotics, devices, and operating room practices. Periprocedural prophylactic antibiotics are administered before neurosurgical device procedures to reduce the risk of associated infection.[4] Several metaanalyses conclude that using periprocedural antibiotics can reduce CSF shunt infection incidence by 50%.[64,65] The antibiotic should be given within 60 minutes before incision to achieve appropriate tissue concentrations. Although it has been common practice to continue prophylactic antibiotics 24 to 48 hours after surgery, guidelines support the use of single-dose prophylaxis.[66,67]

Antibiotic-impregnated catheters for CSF shunts and drains are a relatively recent innovation in neurosurgery that are an additional way to decrease the risk of neurologic device infections. The catheters are typically impregnated with rifampin plus clindamycin or minocycline.[4] The use of antibiotic-impregnated catheters compared with catheters without antibiotics decreases the incidence of CSF shunt and CSF drain infections and decreases hospital expenses.[68–71] Another study found that the time until infection was greater with antibiotic-impregnated catheters compared with the group with a standard CSF drain.[72] Given these data, use of antibiotic-impregnated catheters is recommended for CSF drain or CSF shunt procedures.

The data evaluating the continuation of antibiotics while EVDs or LDs remain in place is currently conflicting. A few studies have found no decrease in the incidence of EVD-associated ventriculitis with prolonged systemic antibiotic therapy.[73,74] However, other studies have found that continuing prophylactic antibiotics while the EVD remains in place is beneficial.[75] Therefore, the use of prophylactic antibiotics to prevent ventriculitis while an EVD or LD is in place remains an area of controversy.

The suggestion of fixed interval exchange of EVDs to prevent infection is not supported by current studies. As discussed elsewhere in this article, a longer duration of EVD placement increases the risk of EVD-associated ventriculitis. Prophylactic EVD exchange was recommended to decrease this risk. However, fixed catheter exchange every 5 days does not decrease the incidence of CSF infection.[76,77] Although the exchange of EVDs does not decrease the risk of infection, removing the EVD as soon as clinically indicated is the optimal strategy to decrease the incidence of EVD-associated infections.

In addition to the neurologic device–specific recommendations made herein, health care providers should also strictly adhere to established guidelines to prevent all surgical site infections.[67] Appropriate infection control recommendations include hand hygiene and the use of gloves and other barrier devices including masks, caps, gowns, drapes, and shoe covers by all personnel in the room. In addition, an approved skin antiseptic agent should be applied according to manufacturer recommendations. Preoperative hair removal increases the risk of surgical site infection.[78] However, if hair removal is absolute necessary, surgical personnel should use clippers or depilatory agents as opposed to razors outside of the operating room.[79,80] Recommended surgical practices include gentle traction, effective hemostasis, removal of devitalized tissues, obliteration of dead space, irrigation of tissues with saline to avoid excessive drying, wound closure without tension, and judicious use of closed suction drains.[79] The prevention of surgical site infections requires a multifactorial approach and adherence from all health care providers preoperatively, perioperatively, and postoperatively.

SUMMARY

Infection is an important complication of neurosurgical devices including shunts, drains, and implanted electrodes. Diagnosis of infections can be challenging because clinical presentations are variable, traditional CSF parameters are unreliable, and CSF cultures are not always positive. Managing infections typically requires a multidisciplinary team approach that includes treatment with antibiotics, debridement, and removal of infected devices.

REFERENCES

1. Blount JP, Campbell JA, Haines SJ. Complications in ventricular cerebrospinal fluid shunting. Neurosurg Clin N Am 1993;4(4):633–56.
2. Kestle JR, Garton HJ, Whitehead WE, et al. Management of shunt infections: a multicenter pilot study. J Neurosurg 2006;105(3 Suppl):177–81.
3. Winn HR, Youmans JR. Youmans & Winn Neurological Surgery. Vol 1. 7th edition. Philadelphia: Elsevier; 2017. p. 1638–43.
4. Tunkel AR, Hasbun R, Bhimraj A, et al. 2017 Infectious Diseases Society of America's clinical practice guidelines for healthcare-associated ventriculitis and meningitis. Clin Infect Dis 2017. https://doi.org/10.1093/cid/ciw861.
5. Simon TD, Butler J, Whitlock KB, et al. Risk factors for first cerebrospinal fluid shunt infection: findings from a multi-center prospective cohort study. J Pediatr 2014;164(6):1462–1468 e2.
6. Borgbjerg BM, Gjerris F, Albeck MJ, et al. Risk of infection after cerebrospinal fluid shunt: an analysis of 884 first-time shunts. Acta Neurochir (Wien) 1995; 136(1–2):1–7.
7. McGirt MJ, Zaas A, Fuchs HE, et al. Risk factors for pediatric ventriculoperitoneal shunt infection and predictors of infectious pathogens. Clin Infect Dis 2003;36(7): 858–62.
8. van de Beek D, Drake JM, Tunkel AR. Nosocomial bacterial meningitis. N Engl J Med 2010;362(2):146–54.
9. Vinchon M, Dhellemmes P. Cerebrospinal fluid shunt infection: risk factors and long-term follow-up. Childs Nerv Syst 2006;22(7):692–7.
10. Wang KW, Chang WN, Shih TY, et al. Infection of cerebrospinal fluid shunts: causative pathogens, clinical features, and outcomes. Jpn J Infect Dis 2004;57(2): 44–8.
11. Shapiro S, Boaz J, Kleiman M, et al. Origin of organisms infecting ventricular shunts. Neurosurgery 1988;22(5):868–72.
12. Kanev PM, Sheehan JM. Reflections on shunt infection. Pediatr Neurosurg 2003; 39(6):285–90.
13. Kulkarni AV, Drake JM, Lamberti-Pasculli M. Cerebrospinal fluid shunt infection: a prospective study of risk factors. J Neurosurg 2001;94(2):195–201.
14. Conen A, Walti LN, Merlo A, et al. Characteristics and treatment outcome of cerebrospinal fluid shunt-associated infections in adults: a retrospective analysis over an 11-year period. Clin Infect Dis 2008;47(1):73–82.

15. Vinchon M, Lemaitre MP, Vallee L, et al. Late shunt infection: incidence, pathogenesis, and therapeutic implications. Neuropediatrics 2002;33(4):169–73.
16. Faillace WJ. A no-touch technique protocol to diminish cerebrospinal fluid shunt infection. Surg Neurol 1995;43(4):344–50.
17. Vinchon M, Baroncini M, Laurent T, et al. Bowel perforation caused by peritoneal shunt catheters: diagnosis and treatment. Neurosurgery 2006;58(1 Suppl): ONS76–82 [discussion: ONS76-82].
18. Thompson TP, Albright AL. Propionibacterium [correction of Proprionibacterium] acnes infections of cerebrospinal fluid shunts. Childs Nerv Syst 1998;14(8): 378–80.
19. Forgacs P, Geyer CA, Freidberg SR. Characterization of chemical meningitis after neurological surgery. Clin Infect Dis 2001;32(2):179–85.
20. Nigrovic LE, Malley R, Macias CG, et al. Effect of antibiotic pretreatment on cerebrospinal fluid profiles of children with bacterial meningitis. Pediatrics 2008; 122(4):726–30.
21. Banks JT, Bharara S, Tubbs RS, et al. Polymerase chain reaction for the rapid detection of cerebrospinal fluid shunt or ventriculostomy infections. Neurosurgery 2005;57(6):1237–43 [discussion: 1237–43].
22. Forward KR, Fewer HD, Stiver HG. Cerebrospinal fluid shunt infections. A review of 35 infections in 32 patients. J Neurosurg 1983;59(3):389–94.
23. Ferreira NP, Otta GM, do Amaral LL, et al. Imaging aspects of pyogenic infections of the central nervous system. Top Magn Reson Imaging 2005;16(2):145–54.
24. Schreffler RT, Schreffler AJ, Wittler RR. Treatment of cerebrospinal fluid shunt infections: a decision analysis. Pediatr Infect Dis J 2002;21(7):632–6.
25. Whitehead WE, Kestle JR. The treatment of cerebrospinal fluid shunt infections. Results from a practice survey of the American society of pediatric neurosurgeons. Pediatr Neurosurg 2001;35(4):205–10.
26. Pelegrin I, Lora-Tamayo J, Gomez-Junyent J, et al. Management of ventriculoperitoneal shunt infections in adults: analysis of risk factors associated with treatment failure. Clin Infect Dis 2017;64(8):989–97.
27. Wen DY, Bottini AG, Hall WA, et al. Infections in neurologic surgery. The intraventricular use of antibiotics. Neurosurg Clin N Am 1992;3(2):343–54.
28. Yogev R. Cerebrospinal fluid shunt infections: a personal view. Pediatr Infect Dis 1985;4(2):113–8.
29. James HE, Walsh JW, Wilson HD, et al. Prospective randomized study of therapy in cerebrospinal fluid shunt infection. Neurosurgery 1980;7(5):459–63.
30. Lozier AP, Sciacca RR, Romagnoli MF, et al. Ventriculostomy-related infections: a critical review of the literature. Neurosurgery 2002;51(1):170–81 [discussion: 181–72].
31. Leverstein-van Hall MA, Hopmans TE, van der Sprenkel JW, et al. A bundle approach to reduce the incidence of external ventricular and lumbar drain-related infections. J Neurosurg 2010;112(2):345–53.
32. Sundbarg G, Nordstrom CH, Soderstrom S. Complications due to prolonged ventricular fluid pressure recording. Br J Neurosurg 1988;2(4):485–95.
33. Lyke KE, Obasanjo OO, Williams MA, et al. Ventriculitis complicating use of intraventricular catheters in adult neurosurgical patients. Clin Infect Dis 2001;33(12): 2028–33.
34. Mayhall CG, Archer NH, Lamb VA, et al. Ventriculostomy-related infections. A prospective epidemiologic study. N Engl J Med 1984;310(9):553–9.

35. Governale LS, Fein N, Logsdon J, et al. Techniques and complications of external lumbar drainage for normal pressure hydrocephalus. Neurosurgery 2008;63(4 Suppl 2):379–84 [discussion: 384].

36. Stenehjem E, Armstrong WS. Central nervous system device infections. Infect Dis Clin North Am 2012;26(1):89–110.

37. Korinek AM. Risk factors for neurosurgical site infections after craniotomy: a prospective multicenter study of 2944 patients. The French Study Group of Neurosurgical Infections, the SEHP, and the C-CLIN Paris-Nord. Service epidemiologie hygiene et prevention. Neurosurgery 1997;41(5):1073–9 [discussion: 1079–81].

38. Korinek AM, Golmard JL, Elcheick A, et al. Risk factors for neurosurgical site infections after craniotomy: a critical reappraisal of antibiotic prophylaxis on 4,578 patients. Br J Neurosurg 2005;19(2):155–62.

39. Odio C, McCracken GH Jr, Nelson JD. CSF shunt infections in pediatrics. A seven-year experience. Am J Dis Child 1984;138(12):1103–8.

40. Walti LN, Conen A, Coward J, et al. Characteristics of infections associated with external ventricular drains of cerebrospinal fluid. J Infect 2013;66(5):424–31.

41. Schade RP, Schinkel J, Visser LG, et al. Bacterial meningitis caused by the use of ventricular or lumbar cerebrospinal fluid catheters. J Neurosurg 2005;102(2):229–34.

42. Muttaiyah S, Ritchie S, Upton A, et al. Clinical parameters do not predict infection in patients with external ventricular drains: a retrospective observational study of daily cerebrospinal fluid analysis. J Med Microbiol 2008;57(Pt 2):207–9.

43. Meredith FT, Phillips HK, Reller LB. Clinical utility of broth cultures of cerebrospinal fluid from patients at risk for shunt infections. J Clin Microbiol 1997;35(12):3109–11.

44. Pfausler B, Beer R, Engelhardt K, et al. Cell index–a new parameter for the early diagnosis of ventriculostomy (external ventricular drainage)-related ventriculitis in patients with intraventricular hemorrhage? Acta Neurochir (Wien) 2004;146(5):477–81.

45. Wong GK, Poon WS, Ip M. Use of ventricular cerebrospinal fluid lactate measurement to diagnose cerebrospinal fluid infection in patients with intraventricular haemorrhage. J Clin Neurosci 2008;15(6):654–5.

46. Deutch S, Dahlberg D, Hedegaard J, et al. Diagnosis of ventricular drainage-related bacterial meningitis by broad-range real-time polymerase chain reaction. Neurosurgery 2007;61(2):306–11 [discussion: 311–2].

47. Pfisterer W, Muhlbauer M, Czech T, et al. Early diagnosis of external ventricular drainage infection: results of a prospective study. J Neurol Neurosurg Psychiatry 2003;74(7):929–32.

48. Schade RP, Schinkel J, Roelandse FW, et al. Lack of value of routine analysis of cerebrospinal fluid for prediction and diagnosis of external drainage-related bacterial meningitis. J Neurosurg 2006;104(1):101–8.

49. Omar AS, ElShawarby A, Singh R. Early monitoring of ventriculostomy-related infections with procalcitonin in patients with ventricular drains. J Clin Monit Comput 2015;29(6):759–65.

50. Berger C, Schwarz S, Schaebitz WR, et al. Serum procalcitonin in cerebral ventriculitis. Crit Care Med 2002;30(8):1778–81.

51. Martinez R, Gaul C, Buchfelder M, et al. Serum procalcitonin monitoring for differential diagnosis of ventriculitis in adult intensive care patients. Intensive Care Med 2002;28(2):208–10.

52. The management of neurosurgical patients with postoperative bacterial or aseptic meningitis or external ventricular drain-associated ventriculitis. Infection in neurosurgery working party of the British society for antimicrobial chemotherapy. Br J Neurosurg 2000;14(1):7–12.

53. Ziai WC, Lewin JJ 3rd. Improving the role of intraventricular antimicrobial agents in the management of meningitis. Curr Opin Neurol 2009;22(3):277–82.

54. Pfausler B, Haring HP, Kampfl A, et al. Cerebrospinal fluid (CSF) pharmacokinetics of intraventricular vancomycin in patients with staphylococcal ventriculitis associated with external CSF drainage. Clin Infect Dis 1997;25(3):733–5.

55. Raad I, Hanna H, Maki D. Intravascular catheter-related infections: advances in diagnosis, prevention, and management. Lancet Infect Dis 2007;7(10):645–57.

56. Beer R, Lackner P, Pfausler B, et al. Nosocomial ventriculitis and meningitis in neurocritical care patients. J Neurol 2008;255(11):1617–24.

57. Fily F, Haegelen C, Tattevin P, et al. Deep brain stimulation hardware-related infections: a report of 12 cases and review of the literature. Clin Infect Dis 2011; 52(8):1020–3.

58. Gorgulho A, Juillard C, Uslan DZ, et al. Infection following deep brain stimulator implantation performed in the conventional versus magnetic resonance imaging-equipped operating room. J Neurosurg 2009;110(2):239–46.

59. Sillay KA, Larson PS, Starr PA. Deep brain stimulator hardware-related infections: incidence and management in a large series. Neurosurgery 2008;62(2):360–6 [discussion: 366–7].

60. Oh MY, Abosch A, Kim SH, et al. Long-term hardware-related complications of deep brain stimulation. Neurosurgery 2002;50(6):1268–74 [discussion: 1274–6].

61. Vergani F, Landi A, Pirillo D, et al. Surgical, medical, and hardware adverse events in a series of 141 patients undergoing subthalamic deep brain stimulation for Parkinson disease. World Neurosurg 2010;73(4):338–44.

62. Merello M, Cammarota A, Leiguarda R, et al. Delayed intracerebral electrode infection after bilateral STN implantation for Parkinson's disease. Case report. Mov Disord 2001;16(1):168–70.

63. Tronnier VM, Staubert A, Hahnel S, et al. Magnetic resonance imaging with implanted neurostimulators: an in vitro and in vivo study. Neurosurgery 1999; 44(1):118–25 [discussion: 125–6].

64. Haines SJ, Walters BC. Antibiotic prophylaxis for cerebrospinal fluid shunts: a metanalysis. Neurosurgery 1994;34(1):87–92.

65. Langley JM, LeBlanc JC, Drake J, et al. Efficacy of antimicrobial prophylaxis in placement of cerebrospinal fluid shunts: meta-analysis. Clin Infect Dis 1993; 17(1):98–103.

66. Bratzler DW, Dellinger EP, Olsen KM, et al. Clinical practice guidelines for antimicrobial prophylaxis in surgery. Am J Health Syst Pharm 2013;70(3):195–283.

67. Berríos-Torres SI, Umscheid CA, Bratzler DW, et al. Centers for disease control and prevention guideline for the prevention of surgical site infection, 2017. JAMA Surg 2017;152(8):784–91.

68. Attenello FJ, Garces-Ambrossi GL, Zaidi HA, et al. Hospital costs associated with shunt infections in patients receiving antibiotic-impregnated shunt catheters versus standard shunt catheters. Neurosurgery 2010;66(2):284–9 [discussion: 289].

69. Parker SL, Anderson WN, Lilienfeld S, et al. Cerebrospinal shunt infection in patients receiving antibiotic-impregnated versus standard shunts. J Neurosurg Pediatr 2011;8(3):259–65.

70. Thomas R, Lee S, Patole S, et al. Antibiotic-impregnated catheters for the prevention of CSF shunt infections: a systematic review and meta-analysis. Br J Neurosurg 2012;26(2):175–84.
71. Parker SL, McGirt MJ, Murphy JA, et al. Comparative effectiveness of antibiotic-impregnated shunt catheters in the treatment of adult and pediatric hydrocephalus: analysis of 12,589 consecutive cases from 287 US hospital systems. J Neurosurg 2015;122(2):443–8.
72. Muttaiyah S, Ritchie S, John S, et al. Efficacy of antibiotic-impregnated external ventricular drain catheters. J Clin Neurosci 2010;17(3):296–8.
73. Alleyne CH Jr, Hassan M, Zabramski JM. The efficacy and cost of prophylactic and perioprocedural antibiotics in patients with external ventricular drains. Neurosurgery 2000;47(5):1124–7 [discussion: 1127–9].
74. Murphy RK, Liu B, Srinath A, et al. No additional protection against ventriculitis with prolonged systemic antibiotic prophylaxis for patients treated with antibiotic-coated external ventricular drains. J Neurosurg 2015;122(5):1120–6.
75. Sonabend AM, Korenfeld Y, Crisman C, et al. Prevention of ventriculostomy-related infections with prophylactic antibiotics and antibiotic-coated external ventricular drains: a systematic review. Neurosurgery 2011;68(4):996–1005.
76. Holloway KL, Barnes T, Choi S, et al. Ventriculostomy infections: the effect of monitoring duration and catheter exchange in 584 patients. J Neurosurg 1996; 85(3):419–24.
77. Wong GK, Poon WS, Wai S, et al. Failure of regular external ventricular drain exchange to reduce cerebrospinal fluid infection: result of a randomised controlled trial. J Neurol Neurosurg Psychiatry 2002;73(6):759–61.
78. Lefebvre A, Saliou P, Lucet JC, et al. Preoperative hair removal and surgical site infections: network meta-analysis of randomized controlled trials. J Hosp Infect 2015;91(2):100–8.
79. Global guidelines for the prevention of surgical site infection. 2016. Available at: https://www.ncbi.nlm.nih.gov/pubmedhealth/PMH0095752/pdf/PubMedHealth_PMH0095752.pdf. Accessed December 20, 2017.
80. Anderson DJ, Podgorny K, Berrios-Torres SI, et al. Strategies to prevent surgical site infections in acute care hospitals: 2014 update. Infect Control Hosp Epidemiol 2014;35(6):605–27.

Breast Implant Infections
An Update

Tahaniyat Lalani, MBBS, MHS

KEYWORDS

- Augmentation mammoplasty • Breast reconstruction • Breast implant infection
- Breast implant removal • Gram-positive pathogens

KEY POINTS

- Postmastectomy implantation is associated with a higher risk of infection compared with breast augmentation alone.
- The timing of breast implant infections can be divided into acute onset (within 6 weeks after surgery), subacute onset (within a few months of surgery), or late-onset infections (more than 6 months after surgery). Most infections are caused by gram-positive pathogens, such as coagulase-negative staphylococci, Cutibacterium species, *Staphylococcus aureus*, and streptococci.
- Acute infections are usually associated with fever and breast pain, erythema, and drainage. Subacute infections may present with chronic pain, persistent drainage, failed healing of the incision site, or migration of the implant.
- Diagnosis of implant infections is generally clinical (ie, based on the presenting signs and symptoms). Depending on the severity of infection, patients are started on empiric intravenous or oral antibiotics and closely monitored for signs of improvement.
- Implant removal is often necessary for cure, particularly in patients with systemic toxicity, failure to improve, or worsening on empiric antibiotics or atypical mycobacterial and fungal infections. Culture data should be used to guide antibiotic therapy.

BACKGROUND

Augmentation mammoplasty with prosthetic breast implantation is a common surgical procedure used for breast enlargement, for correction of asymmetries, or for reconstruction after mastectomy. Two types of breast prostheses are currently available in the United States: silicone gel implants and saline implants. Silicone implants, consisting of a silicone polymer shell filled with silicone gel, are preferred for augmentation because they provide a more natural appearance and feel. Saline implants offer the

Disclosure Statement: No conflicts or disclosures to declare.
Preventive Medicine and Biostatistics, Uniformed Services University of the Health Science, 4301 Jones Bridge Road, Bethesda, MD 20814, USA
E-mail address: tlalani@idcrp.org

Infect Dis Clin N Am 32 (2018) 877–884
https://doi.org/10.1016/j.idc.2018.06.007
0891-5520/18/Published by Elsevier Inc.

id.theclinics.com

advantage of a smaller incision because they are inserted as empty shells and filled to the appropriate volume by adding the saline solution.

Breast implants in reconstruction following mastectomy are usually placed under the pectoralis major muscle (submuscular) either immediately after mastectomy (1-stage) or following the use of a tissue expander (2-stage). The prosthetic tissue expander is placed under the muscle through the mastectomy incision and filled gradually through a subcutaneous port using weekly saline injections until the proper volume is achieved. At the next stage, the expander is removed and an implant is placed in the expanded pocket. An acellular dermal matrix, composed of extracellular matrix structures of bovine, porcine, or human cadaveric origin, or synthetic mesh can be used as an adjuncts to tissue expanders for shaping the reconstructive breast and anchoring the implant to the chest wall. Non-reconstructive augmentation for cosmetic purposes is usually performed through an inframammary or periareolar incision with placement of the implant in either the subglandular or the submuscular position.

Aside from prosthetic implant infections, additional surgery or removal of implant is often required for complications, such as capsular contractures (10-year incidence: 9.2% for augmentation and 14.5% for reconstruction), implant rupture (10-year incidence: 9%), implant malposition, asymmetry, wrinkling, or seromas (<5%). Periodic MRIs of breast implants are recommended to determine if implant rupture has occurred.

EPIDEMIOLOGY AND RISK FACTORS

Breast implant infections usually present in a bimodal fashion: during the acute postoperative period (6 days to 6 weeks after surgery) or with subacute or late onset (more than 6 weeks to months after surgery). In a worldwide survey conducted in 1970, the incidence of early and late-onset infections in 10,941 women who underwent breast augmentation was 1.7% and 0.8%, respectively. The overall incidence of implant infections was 2.5%.[1] Lower rates of infection and an equal distribution of early- and late-onset infections have been reported in recent studies.[2,3]

Risk factors for breast implant infections include the patient's underlying clinical comorbidities as well as intraoperative and postoperative factors. Women undergoing reconstructive surgery following mastectomy, axillary dissection,[4] chemotherapy,[5] or radiation therapy are at significantly increased risk of infection, up to 10 times higher than women undergoing nonreconstructive augmentation for cosmetic purposes.[6–8] The increased risk of infection is likely due to preexisting tissue scarring, ischemia, and delayed wound healing. Infection is less likely to occur with delayed placement of the implant in postmastectomy patients, as part of a 2-stage procedure.[1,9] Other risk factors for breast implant infection include obesity, diabetes mellitus, renal failure, active skin disorders, and tobacco use.[10,11]

Intraoperative risk factors, such as surgical technique and surgical environment (eg, leading to hematoma or ischemia during surgery), lymph node dissection, and contamination of the implant or saline, have been implicated in reports of breast implant infections. No difference in the risk of infection between silicone and saline implants has been reported. However, the use of acellular dermal matrix as an adjunct to the placement of an implant or tissue expander is associated with higher rates of seroma formation and surgical site infections. In one meta-analysis, acellular dermal matrix use was associated with infection (odds ratio [OR] = 1.47, 95% confidence interval [CI] 1.04–2.06) but not explantation (OR 1.37, 95% CI: 0.89–2.11). Surgical drains were associated with a 5-fold increase in risk in one study, but no increase in risk was demonstrated in a subsequent report.[12,13] Potential contamination of the implant by the endogenous flora of the nipple or breast ducts with the periareolar or transareolar approaches has been proposed as a theoretic risk.[8]

Late-onset infections, occurring months to years after implantation, usually occur due to seeding of the implant from a remote source.

MICROBIOLOGY AND PATHOGENESIS

Contamination of the breast implant with endogenous gram-positive organisms gaining access to deeper breast tissue during surgery, such as coagulase-negative staphylococci, *Cutibacterium* species, *Staphylococcus aureus*, and streptococci, is responsible for most early-onset infections. In a single-center, retrospective review conducted at a referral center in south France, gram-negative bacilli (*Pseudomonas aeruginosa* in particular) were noted to be the second leading cause of microbiologically confirmed breast implant infections after *S aureus*.[3] Rarely, infections due to contamination of the implant or saline or skin marking solution (eg, nontuberculous mycobacteria, Curvularia,[14] gram-negative bacteria such Pseudomonas, and anaerobes[15]), or due to hematogenous seeding of the implant, have been reported.[8,16–19] *Mycobacterium fortuitum* is most often associated with breast implant infection, but multiple other nontuberculous mycobacteria, including *Mycobacterium avium*, *Mycobacterium abscessus*, and *Mycobacterium chelonae*, have been implicated.[15,20–31]

The pathogenesis of breast implant infections involves an initial phase of adhesion of bacteria to other cells and the implant surface using cell wall proteins, conversion to a sessile form, and secretion of an extracellular polymeric substance, which forms a barrier between the bacterial microcolonies and extracellular environment.[32] In animal models, the presence of a subcutaneous foreign body reduces the minimal inoculum of *S aureus* required to cause infection by a factor of more than 100,000, to as little as 100 colony-forming units (CFU). Ultimately, a mature biofilm is formed that is characterized by channels surrounding macrocolonies, allowing for the distribution of nutrients and signaling molecules. Bacteria embedded in biofilms are often resistant to killing by antimicrobials despite in vitro susceptibility, therefore necessitating the removal of the foreign body for eradication of the infection. The lack of a microcirculation in the implanted material and impaired neutrophil function further enhance the susceptibility to infection.[33–37]

Clinical Manifestations

Breast implant infections usually present in a bimodal fashion. Early-onset infections occur during the first 6 weeks after surgery and are associated with both local and systemic signs of infection, such as fever, breast pain, erythema, and purulent fluid or drainage at the site of the incision. Rarely, toxic shock syndrome can complicate an early implant infection due to *S aureus* or streptococci, manifesting within hours or days of implantation. In a review by Holm and colleagues,[38] the median duration between surgery and toxic shock syndrome was 4 days, although symptom onset within 12 to 24 hours after surgery has also been reported.[39–46] Toxic shock syndrome typically presents with signs of sepsis (such as fever, rash, nausea, vomiting, diarrhea, hypotension, and multiorgan system failure) and a lack of signs of infection at the operative site. Therefore, a high index of suspicion is needed to diagnose patients presenting with sepsis soon after implant placement, because prompt removal of the prosthesis is imperative to patient survival.

An important differential diagnosis to consider in patients undergoing implantation using acellular dermal matrix is the "red breast syndrome," a self-limited, painless, blanching erythema of the breast overlying the acellular matrix that presents in the first few weeks following surgery. Alloderm, in particular, is associated with the syndrome of uncertain cause. The erythema typically resolves within a few weeks or months without treatment and is not associated with other signs of cellulitis such as fever, pain, or leukocytosis.[47]

Subacute infections due to indolent bacteria, such as coagulase-negative staphylococcus and *Cutibacterium* spp, present several months after implantation with focal symptoms, such as a nonhealing surgical site, incisional drainage, dehiscence, or extrusion of the implant. Nontuberculous mycobacterial infections are important to consider in patients with acute or subacute symptoms with a serous or seropurulent drainage that is culture-negative on routine bacterial cultures.

Late-onset infections occur due to hematogenous seeding of the implant with gram-positive or gram-negative organisms and present with dehiscence, drainage, cellulitis, or a periprosthetic abscess.[48] A case series of late-onset *Serratia marcescens*–associated implant infections linked the infection to the repeated use of an individual saline bag used for implant expansion, which was extrinsically contaminated due to poor hand hygiene and breaks in aseptic technique at the time of implant expansion.[49]

The role of infection and biofilm formation in capsular contractures, a common late-onset complication of breast implants, is unproven, although animal models and small case series report isolating bacteria in patients with capsular contractures. In a prospective, single-center study at the Mayo Clinic, breast implants removed for reasons other than infection underwent vortexing/sonication procedure followed by semiquantitative culture. Nine of 27 (33%) implants removed due to significant capsular contracture had $\geq$20 CFU bacteria/10 mL sonicate fluid versus 1 (5%) of 18, removed for reasons other than capsular contracture.[50]

Diagnosis

Diagnosis of breast implant infection is largely clinical, based on local and systemic symptoms of infection. As noted above, implant infections should be considered in patients presenting with toxic shock syndrome who have recently undergone implantation. Patients with systemic signs of infection, such as fever, hypotension, or sepsis, should have blood cultures drawn to assess for concomitant bacteremia. Differentiation from red breast syndrome, cellulitis, and superficial surgical site infection is also important for management. Superficial swabbing of draining fluid at the surgical site is not useful due to contamination with skin flora. Ultrasound imaging and guided aspiration are recommended in cases with a suspected periprosthetic fluid collection, and any aspirated fluid should be sent for standard aerobic and anaerobic bacteria, fungal, and mycobacterial cultures. Any debrided tissue and removed implants should be examined histopathologically and sent for culture as noted above.

Treatment

Management of breast implant infection usually entails prompt initiation of empiric antibiotic therapy, followed by a period of a few days of close observation to determine if implant removal or salvage is appropriate. Implant removal is often necessary to achieve cure especially in infections due to virulent pathogens, such as *S aureus* or fungi, or if a rapid improvement in signs of infection is not observed following antibiotic therapy. In subacute cases or in surgical site infections without signs of systemic toxicity, an oral empiric regimen of antibiotics for 48 hours pending culture data is appropriate. In such cases, clinical deterioration or lack of response warrants hospitalization for further evaluation and parenteral antibiotic therapy.

In a retrospective review of patients with breast implant infections treated with medical therapy alone, 8 patients with mild infection (defined as warmth, swelling, or cellulitis without drainage) were treated with oral antibiotics, and all responded without requiring removal of the implant. Two of 4 patients with persistent swelling despite antibiotic therapy, purulent drainage, systemic signs of infection, or atypical organisms, such as gram-negative rods or mycobacteria, were salvaged with antibiotic therapy alone.[51]

Empiric antibiotic regimens should include coverage for methicillin-resistant S aureus and coagulase-negative staphylococcus and gram-negative bacteria. Patients with systemic signs of infection are usually started on intravenous therapy such as Vancomycin (30–60 mg/kg per day in two to three divided doses) and Piperacillin/tazobactam (3.375 g every 6 hours). If rapid improvement in symptoms is noted within 1 to 2 days, patients can be switched to suitable oral alternatives, such as clindamycin, trimethoprim-sulfamethoxazole, linezolid, and/or ciprofloxacin. When possible, antimicrobials should be tailored to target pathogens identified on culture.

Duration of antibiotic therapy

Superficial surgical site infections limited to a mild cellulitis without a periprosthetic fluid collection or drainage and without systemic signs can be treated with 10 to 14 days of oral antibiotic therapy and close monitoring without implant removal.

Patients undergoing debridement and implant removal are treated with 10 to 14 days of antibiotics, guided by operative cultures. A longer duration of therapy is needed for atypical mycobacterial infections. Reimplantation may be considered following completion of antibiotic therapy and no recurrence of symptoms following cessation of antibiotics. Some experts recommend delaying reimplantation until 4 to 6 months or more after completion of antibiotic therapy. In a case series of 9 patients undergoing secondary implant placement, one patient developed a recurrent infection requiring explantation.[52]

Treatment of implant infections with debridement and retention of implant or "one-stage replacement" are not recommended. Reports of successful salvage using this strategy are limited to small case series with insufficient long-term outcome data.[53–55]

Prevention

Adherence with preoperative, intraoperative, and postoperative guidelines by the Centers for Disease Control and Prevention and other agencies for prevention of surgical site infections is key for preventing surgical site infections during implantation.[56] Although perioperative antibiotic prophylaxis with cefazolin (1–2 g intravenous given within 60 minutes before the surgical incision) is widely used by surgeons at the time of implantation, this is not supported by high-quality evidence or expert guidelines.[57–59] Routine antimicrobial prophylaxis for "clean" procedures such as breast surgery is not recommended, although some experts recommend prophylaxis for procedures that involve placement of prosthetic material in patients with risk factors for infection, such as diabetes mellitus, obesity, tobacco use, coexisting infections elsewhere, known colonization with microorganisms, and immunocompromising conditions.[60] Similarly, there is limited evidence to support the use of topical antimicrobials and antiseptics for irrigation of the surgical pocket at the time of implantation to prevent surgical site infections and capsular contractures.[12,61] Patients with existing implants do not need antibiotic prophylaxis when undergoing invasive dental procedures.

REFERENCES

1. De Cholnoky T. Augmentation mammaplasty. Survey of complications in 10,941 patients by 265 surgeons. Plast Reconstr Surg 1970;45:573–7.
2. Duteille F, Perrot P, Bacheley MH, et al. Eight-year safety data for round and anatomical silicone gel breast implants. Aesthet Surg J 2017;38(2):151–61.
3. Seng P, Bayle S, Alliez A, et al. The microbial epidemiology of breast implant infections in a regional referral centre for plastic and reconstructive surgery in the south of France. Int J Infect Dis 2015;35:62–6.
4. Nahabedian MY, Tsangaris T, Momen B, et al. Infectious complications following breast reconstruction with expanders and implants. Plast Reconstr Surg 2003; 112:467–76.
5. Vandeweyer E, Deraemaecker R, Nogaret JM, et al. Immediate breast reconstruction with implants and adjuvant chemotherapy: a good option? Acta Chir Belg 2003;103:98–101.
6. Courtiss EH, Goldwyn RM, Anastasi GW. The fate of breast implants with infections around them. Plast Reconstr Surg 1979;63:812–6.
7. Gabriel SE, Woods JE, O'Fallon WM, et al. Complications leading to surgery after breast implantation. N Engl J Med 1997;336:677–82.
8. Pittet B, Montandon D, Pittet D. Infection in breast implants. Lancet Infect Dis 2005;5:94–106.
9. Baker JlJW. Augmentation mammaplasty. In: Owsley JE, editor. Symposium of aesthetic surgery of the breast: Proceedings of the Symposium of the Educational Foundation of the American Society of Plastic and Reconstructive Surgeons and the American Society for Aesthetic Plastic Surgery, in Scottsdale, AZ, November 23-26, 1975. St Louis, MO: Mosby; 1978. p. 256–63.
10. Kato H, Nakagami G, Iwahira Y, et al. Risk factors and risk scoring tool for infection during tissue expansion in tissue expander and implant breast reconstruction. Breast J 2013;19:618–26.
11. Mlodinow AS, Ver Halen JP, Lim S, et al. Predictors of readmission after breast reconstruction: a multi-institutional analysis of 5012 patients. Ann Plast Surg 2013;71:335–41.
12. Araco A, Gravante G, Araco F, et al. Infections of breast implants in aesthetic breast augmentations: a single-center review of 3,002 patients. Aesthetic Plast Surg 2007;31:325–9.
13. McCarthy CM, Mehrara BJ, Riedel E, et al. Predicting complications following expander/implant breast reconstruction: an outcomes analysis based on preoperative clinical risk. Plast Reconstr Surg 2008;121:1886–92.
14. Kainer MA, Keshavarz H, Jensen BJ, et al. Saline-filled breast implant contamination with Curvularia species among women who underwent cosmetic breast augmentation. J Infect Dis 2005;192:170–7.
15. Safranek TJ, Jarvis WR, Carson LA, et al. Mycobacterium chelonae wound infections after plastic surgery employing contaminated gentian violet skin-marking solution. N Engl J Med 1987;317:197–201.
16. Brand KG. Infection of mammary prostheses: a survey and the question of prevention. Ann Plast Surg 1993;30:289–95.
17. Gibney J. The long-term results of tissue expansion for breast reconstruction. Clin Plast Surg 1987;14:509–18.
18. Ablaza VJ, LaTrenta GS. Late infection of a breast prosthesis with Enterococcus avium. Plast Reconstr Surg 1998;102:227–30.

19. Petit F, Maladry D, Werther JR, et al. Late infection of breast implant, complication of colonic perforation. Review of the literature. Role of preventive treatment. Ann Chir Plast Esthet 1998;43:559–62 [in French].

20. Macadam SA, Mehling BM, Fanning A, et al. Nontuberculous mycobacterial breast implant infections. Plast Reconstr Surg 2007;119:337–44.

21. Vinh DC, Rendina A, Turner R, et al. Breast implant infection with Mycobacterium fortuitum group: report of case and review. J Infect 2006;52:e63–7.

22. Boettcher AK, Bengtson BP, Farber ST, et al. Breast infections with atypical mycobacteria following reduction mammaplasty. Aesthet Surg J 2010;30:542–8.

23. Haiavy J, Tobin H. Mycobacterium fortuitum infection in prosthetic breast implants. Plast Reconstr Surg 2002;109:2124–8.

24. Pereira LH, Sterodimas A. Autologous fat transplantation and delayed silicone implant insertion in a case of Mycobacterium avium breast infection. Aesthetic Plast Surg 2010;34:1–4.

25. Wirth GA, Brenner KA, Sundine MJ. Delayed silicone breast implant infection with Mycobacterium avium-intracellulare. Aesthet Surg J 2007;27:167–71.

26. Feldman EM, Ellsworth W, Yuksel E, et al. Mycobacterium abscessus infection after breast augmentation: a case of contaminated implants? J Plast Reconstr Aesthet Surg 2009;62:e330–2.

27. Jackowe DJ, Murariu D, Parsa NN, et al. Chronic fistulas after breast augmentation secondary to Mycobacterium abscessus. Plast Reconstr Surg 2010;126: 38e–9e.

28. Thibeaut S, Levy PY, Pelletier ML, et al. Mycobacterium conceptionense infection after breast implant surgery, France. Emerg Infect Dis 2010;16:1180–1.

29. Wolfe JM, Moore DF. Isolation of Mycobacterium thermoresistibile following augmentation mammaplasty. J Clin Microbiol 1992;30:1036–8.

30. Padoveze MC, Fortaleza CM, Freire MP, et al. Outbreak of surgical infection caused by non-tuberculous mycobacteria in breast implants in Brazil. J Hosp Infect 2007;67:161–7.

31. Rahav G, Pitlik S, Amitai Z, et al. An outbreak of Mycobacterium jacuzzii infection following insertion of breast implants. Clin Infect Dis 2006;43:823–30.

32. Oliveira WF, Silva PMS, Silva RCS, et al. Staphylococcus aureus and Staphylococcus epidermidis infections on implants. J Hosp Infect 2018;98(2):111–7.

33. Zimmerli W, Waldvogel FA, Vaudaux P, et al. Pathogenesis of foreign body infection: description and characteristics of an animal model. J Infect Dis 1982;146: 487–97.

34. Zimmerli W, Lew PD, Waldvogel FA. Pathogenesis of foreign body infection. Evidence for a local granulocyte defect. J Clin Invest 1984;73:1191–200.

35. Costerton JW, Stewart PS, Greenberg EP. Bacterial biofilms: a common cause of persistent infections. Science 1999;284:1318–22.

36. Donlan RM. Biofilm formation: a clinically relevant microbiological process. Clin Infect Dis 2001;33:1387–92.

37. Vuong C, Gerke C, Somerville GA, et al. Quorum-sensing control of biofilm factors in Staphylococcus epidermidis. J Infect Dis 2003;188:706–18.

38. Holm C, Muhlbauer W. Toxic shock syndrome in plastic surgery patients: case report and review of the literature. Aesthetic Plast Surg 1998;22:180–4.

39. Barnett A, Lavey E, Pearl RM, et al. Toxic shock syndrome from an infected breast prosthesis. Ann Plast Surg 1983;10:408–10.

40. Walker LE, Breiner MJ, Goodman CM. Toxic shock syndrome after explantation of breast implants: a case report and review of the literature. Plast Reconstr Surg 1997;99:875–9.

41. Bartlett P, Reingold AL, Graham DR, et al. Toxic shock syndrome associated with surgical wound infections. JAMA 1982;247:1448–50.

42. Knudsen F, Olesen AS, Hojbjerg T, et al. Toxic shock syndrome. Br Med J (Clin Res Ed) 1981;282:399.

43. Tobin G, Shaw RC, Goodpasture HC. Toxic shock syndrome following breast and nasal surgery. Plast Reconstr Surg 1987;80:111–4.

44. Olesen LL, Ejlertsen T, Nielsen J. Toxic shock syndrome following insertion of breast prostheses. Br J Surg 1991;78:585–6.

45. Poblete JV, Rodgers JA, Wolfort FG. Toxic shock syndrome as a complication of breast prostheses. Plast Reconstr Surg 1995;96:1702–8.

46. Giesecke J, Arnander C. Toxic shock syndrome after augmentation mammaplasty. Ann Plast Surg 1986;17:532–3.

47. Wu PS, Winocour S, Jacobson SR. Red breast syndrome: a review of available literature. Aesthetic Plast Surg 2015;39:227–30.

48. Washer LL, Gutowski K. Breast implant infections. Infect Dis Clin North Am 2012; 26:111–25.

49. Pegues DA, Shireley LA, Riddle CF, et al. Serratia marcescens surgical wound infection following breast reconstruction. Am J Med 1991;91:173S–8S.

50. Del Pozo JL, Tran NV, Petty PM, et al. Pilot study of association of bacteria on breast implants with capsular contracture. J Clin Microbiol 2009;47:1333–7.

51. Spear SL, Howard MA, Boehmler JH, et al. The infected or exposed breast implant: management and treatment strategies. Plast Reconstr Surg 2004;113: 1634–44.

52. Halvorson EG, Disa JJ, Mehrara BJ, et al. Outcome following removal of infected tissue expanders in breast reconstruction: a 10-year experience. Ann Plast Surg 2007;59:131–6.

53. Prince MD, Suber JS, Aya-Ay ML, et al. Prosthesis salvage in breast reconstruction patients with periprosthetic infection and exposure. Plast Reconstr Surg 2012;129:42–8.

54. Bennett SP, Fitoussi AD, Berry MG, et al. Management of exposed, infected implant-based breast reconstruction and strategies for salvage. J Plast Reconstr Aesthet Surg 2011;64:1270–7.

55. Agarwal S, Ettinger RE, Kung TA, et al. Cohort study of immediate implant exchange during acute infection in the setting of breast reconstruction. J Plast Reconstr Aesthet Surg 2017;70:865–70.

56. Berrios-Torres SI, Umscheid CA, Bratzler DW, et al. Centers for disease control and prevention guideline for the prevention of surgical site infection, 2017. JAMA Surg 2017;152:784–91.

57. Phillips BT, Bishawi M, Dagum AB, et al. A systematic review of antibiotic use and infection in breast reconstruction: what is the evidence? Plast Reconstr Surg 2013;131:1–13.

58. Phillips BT, Halvorson EG. Antibiotic prophylaxis following implant-based breast reconstruction: what is the evidence? Plast Reconstr Surg 2016;138:751–7.

59. Hardwicke JT, Bechar J, Skillman JM. Are systemic antibiotics indicated in aesthetic breast surgery? A systematic review of the literature. Plast Reconstr Surg 2013;131:1395–403.

60. Bratzler DW, Dellinger EP, Olsen KM, et al. Clinical practice guidelines for antimicrobial prophylaxis in surgery. Am J Health Syst Pharm 2013;70:195–283.

61. Adams WP Jr, Rios JL, Smith SJ. Enhancing patient outcomes in aesthetic and reconstructive breast surgery using triple antibiotic breast irrigation: six-year prospective clinical study. Plast Reconstr Surg 2006;118:46S–52S.

Urinary Catheter-Associated Infections

Emily K. Shuman, MD[a,b,]*, Carol E. Chenoweth, MD[a,c]

KEYWORDS

- Prevention • Catheter-associated urinary tract infection
- Health care-associated infection • Urinary catheter

KEY POINTS

- Catheter-associated urinary tract infection is common and costly.
- Catheter-associated urinary tract infection is often caused by hospital-based pathogens with a propensity toward antimicrobial resistance.
- Duration of urinary catheterization is the predominant risk for catheter-associated urinary tract infection; limiting placement and early removal can successfully decrease catheter use and catheter-associated urinary tract infection rates.
- Intervention bundles, collaboratives, and hospital leadership engagement are powerful tools for implementing preventive measures for health care-associated infections, including catheter-associated urinary tract infection.

INTRODUCTION

Catheter-associated urinary tract infection (CAUTI) is a common health care-associated infection, with significant impact on clinical outcomes, including duration of hospital stay and cost of care. The Centers for Disease Control and Prevention estimated that 93,300 CAUTIs occurred in US hospitals in 2011.[1] Urinary tract infections (UTIs) account for 12.9% of health care-associated infections and 23% of infections in the intensive care unit (ICU).[1,2] Urinary catheters are associated with the majority of health care-associated UTIs; approximately 70% of UTIs (95% of UTIs occurring in ICUs) develop in patients with urinary catheters.[3] The occurrence of CAUTI increases cost and duration of hospital stay by 4 days.[4,5]

Disclosures: None.
[a] Division of Infectious Diseases, Department of Internal Medicine, Michigan Medicine, F4007 University Hospital South, 1500 East Medical Center Drive, Ann Arbor, MI 48109-5226, USA; [b] Department of Infection Prevention and Epidemiology, Michigan Medicine, 300 North Ingalls Building 8B06, Ann Arbor, MI 48109-5479, USA; [c] Antimicrobial Stewardship Program, Michigan Medicine, F4141 University Hospital South, 1500 East Medical Center Drive, Ann Arbor, MI 48109-5226, USA
* Corresponding author. F4007 University Hospital South, 1500 East Medical Center Drive, Ann Arbor, MI 48109-5226.
E-mail address: emilyks@umich.edu

Infect Dis Clin N Am 32 (2018) 885–897
https://doi.org/10.1016/j.idc.2018.07.002
0891-5520/18/© 2018 Elsevier Inc. All rights reserved.

The majority of CAUTIs, 65% to 70%, are predicted to be preventable.[6] Because of this, the Centers for Medicare and Medicaid Services (CMS) no longer reimburses hospitals for the extra costs of managing a patient with hospital-acquired CAUTI.[7] The CMS also requires, as a condition of participation, that hospitals submit CAUTI rates to the National Healthcare Safety Network (NHSN) and reports CAUTI as a Healthcare Associated Condition on the CMS website. Therefore, prevention of CAUTI has become a priority for most hospitals. This article reviews the epidemiology, risk factors, and pathogenesis of CAUTI, with a focus on prevention.

EPIDEMIOLOGY OF CATHETER-ASSOCIATED URINARY TRACT INFECTION
Descriptive Epidemiology

Rates of CAUTI in US hospitals have decreased significantly over the past few decades, primarily related to increased emphasis on prevention.[8–10] Pooled mean rates of CAUTI in ICUs, reported through the NHSN in 2013, ranged from to 1.3 UTI per 1000 catheter-days in small medical/surgical ICUs to 5.3 UTI per 1000 catheter-days in neurosurgical ICUs.[8] Rates of CAUTI in general care wards were similar, ranging from 0.2 to 3.2 per 1000 catheter-days; the highest rates occurred in hematology and rehabilitation wards.[8,10] CAUTI occurs in pediatric ICUs occur at similar rates of 0 to 3.4 UTI per 1000 catheter-days; these rates may not be decreasing as in other ICUs.[8,11] In a community hospital consortium, rates of CAUTI were found to be similar in ICU and non-ICU care units, but 72% of CAUTIs occurred in non-ICU patients, suggesting that targeted prevention efforts for non-ICU patients may have a significant impact.[12] This finding has been supported by a recent national prevention program, which resulted in reduction of catheter use and CAUTI in non-ICU settings, with minimal change in ICU settings.[10]

Rates of CAUTI reported through the International Nosocomial Infection Control Consortium have been generally higher than those reported through the NHSN. From 2010 to 2015, the CAUTI pooled mean rate for 50 countries was 5.07 UTI per 1000 catheter-days, but rates ranged of 1.66 UTI per 1000 catheter-days in surgical cardiothoracic ICUs to 17.17 UTI per 1000 catheter-days in neurologic ICUs.[13]

Microbial Etiology

The most common pathogens associated with CAUTI are gram-negative bacilli, Enterobacteriaceae and *Pseudomonas spp*, but in the ICU setting, *Candida spp* and *Enterococcus spp* become more prevalent.[14,15] Antimicrobial resistance in CAUTI isolates has risen in recent decades; in summary reports from the NHSN from 2011 to 2014, 20% to 23.8% of *Klebsiella spp* and 12.8% to 16.1% of *Escherichia coli* isolates from patients with CAUTI produced extended-spectrum beta-lactamases. Additionally, approximately 10% of all *Klebsiella spp* isolates from patients with CAUTI during that time period were resistant to carbapenems.[15] Resistance to antimicrobials in CAUTI isolates was even greater in long-term acute care hospitals, where 38.2% and 11.1% of Enterobacteriaceae exhibited extended-spectrum beta-lactamase phenotype and carbapenem resistance, respectively, in 2014.[14] CAUTI isolates from pediatric ICUs and pediatric wards are also showing higher rates of resistance in *E coli*, with 13.1% and 16.5% extended-spectrum beta-lactamase production identified, respectively.[16]

Risk Factors

Duration of catheterization is the most important risk factor for CAUTI, and is the most modifiable.[2,3] Bacteriuria, the precursor of CAUTI, develops at an average rate of 3%

to 10% per day of catheterization. All patients who are catheterized for 1 month will develop bacteriuria; as such, catheterization for longer than 1 month is used as the definition for long-term catheterization.[2] Other modifiable risk factors are associated with health care provider knowledge, skill, and adherence to infection prevention recommendations (**Table 1**). Systemic antimicrobial agents have a protective effect on bacteriuria (relative risk [RR], 2.0–3.9).[2,17]

Table 1 also outlines major host-level risk factors for CAUTI. Females have a shorter urethra and hence higher risk of bacteriuria than males; heavy bacterial colonization of the perineum increases that risk. Other patient factors identified in one or more studies include age greater than 50 years, rapidly fatal underlying illness, nonsurgical disease, hospitalization on an orthopedic or urologic service, catheter insertion after day 6 of hospitalization, catheter insertion outside the operating room, diabetes mellitus, and renal insufficiency (serum creatinine >2 mg/dL) at the time of catheterization.[2,17]

Urinary catheter-associated bloodstream infection is a rare event, occurring in less than 4% of CAUTIs.[18–20] Risk factors for bloodstream infection from a urinary source include male sex, immunosuppressant therapy, history of malignancy, neutropenia, renal disease, cigarette use in the past 5 years, and number of hospital days before bacteriuria infection.[19–22] Prevention strategies for patients at highest risk of bloodstream infection may be incorporated into an overall CAUTI prevention program.

PATHOGENESIS

Most microorganisms causing CAUTI originate from endogenous organisms colonizing the patient's intestinal tract and perineum and enter the bladder by ascending the urethra from the perineum.[23] Two-thirds of these organisms migrate in the biofilm on the external surface of the catheter, whereas one-third of infections are acquired from intraluminal contamination of the collection system from exogenous sources.[23,24] Although most CAUTIs are caused by microorganisms from the patient's own gastrointestinal tract, approximately 15% of episodes of health care-associated bacteriuria occur in clusters from intrahospital transmission from one patient to another.[2,24] Most of these hospital-based outbreaks have been associated with improper hand hygiene by health care personnel.

Humans have innate defense mechanisms, such as length of urethra and urine flow, that prevent most pathogens from entering into the bladder, but urinary catheters interfere with these natural defenses.[2,25] Biofilms, made of clusters of microorganisms and extracellular matrix, deposit on all surfaces of urinary catheters and allow bacterial attachment.[26–28] Biofilms also provide a protective environment from immune cells and antimicrobials and have been found to drive colonization and infection with multidrug-resistant pathogens.[26–28] Microorganisms grow more slowly in biofilms, decreasing the effectiveness of many antimicrobials. Nevertheless, despite slow growth, microorganisms in the biofilm may ascend the catheter to the bladder in 1

Table 1	
Risk factors for catheter-associated urinary tract infection	
Host-Level Risk Factors	**Modifiable Risk Factors**
Female sex	Duration of catheterization (dominant)
Age >50 y	Nonadherence to aseptic catheter care
Severe underlying illness	(ie, opening closed system)
Nonsurgical disease	Lower professional training of inserter
Diabetes mellitus	Catheter insertion outside operating room
Serum creatinine >2 mg/dL	Catheter insertion after 6th day of hospitalization

to 3 days. Typically, the biofilm is composed of 1 type of microorganism, although polymicrobial biofilms are possible.[28]

DIAGNOSIS

The clinical diagnosis of CAUTI remains challenging, because neither bacteriuria or pyuria are reliable indicators of symptomatic UTI, especially in the setting of long-term catheterization, where bacteriuria is universal.[29,30] In addition, urine cultures may grow significant numbers of bacteria if improperly collected and transported.[31,32]

Urine cultures are often collected for inappropriate reasons or as part of a generic fever evaluation, without symptoms referable to the urinary tract.[33–35] In such cases, asymptomatic bacteriuria may be treated inappropriately, even when another source of fever has been identified.[36–38] However, the distinction between asymptomatic versus symptomatic UTI is clinically important, because asymptomatic catheter-associated bacteriuria rarely results in adverse outcomes and treatment is not recommended.[39] Recent antimicrobial stewardship programs have resulted in a decrease in inappropriate urine culture collection and treatment of asymptomatic bacteriuria.[40,41]

SURVEILLANCE

The NHSN has developed surveillance definitions for UTI and CAUTI that allow for standardization and interfacility comparison of infection rates.[42] The definitions distinguish between symptomatic UTI and asymptomatic bacteriuria. To meet criteria for a symptomatic UTI, an adult patient must have at least one sign or symptom (temperature $>38°C$, urinary urgency, urinary frequency, dysuria, suprapubic tenderness, or costovertebral angle pain or tenderness) and a positive urine culture ($\geq 10^5$ colony forming units/mL with no more than 2 species of organisms detected). Symptomatic UTI is considered to be catheter associated if a urinary catheter has been in place for more than 2 days and at least one of the above signs or symptoms is present (with the exception of urgency, frequency, or dysuria if the catheter is still in place). Asymptomatic bacteriuria is defined as a positive urine culture ($\geq 10^5$ colony forming units/mL with no more than 2 species of organisms detected) in the absence of signs or symptoms. One change that was made with recent NHSN surveillance definitions is that *Candida spp* and other yeasts are no longer considered urinary pathogens, and patients with urine cultures growing yeast only are not considered to have a symptomatic UTI.

Surveillance for CAUTI had not been a priority for most hospitals in the past, mostly because of a lack of resources required to perform full hospital surveillance. However, in January 2012, most acute care facilities began reporting CAUTIs from adult and pediatric ICUs to the NHSN to meet the requirements of the CMS Inpatient Prospective Payment System final rule.[43] Beginning in January 2015, acute care hospitals were also required to report CAUTIs from adult and pediatric medical and surgical wards. CAUTI rates are publicly reported on the CMS Hospital Compare website.[44] Some states also have requirements for CAUTI reporting.

Surveillance for CAUTI should be performed using NHSN definitions, and data collection forms using these standardized criteria are available from the NHSN. The incidence of CAUTI is typically expressed as the number of infections per 1000 urinary catheter-days.[45] However, the use of device days as a denominator may mask successful CAUTI prevention efforts, because an overall decrease in catheter use may paradoxically lead to higher CAUTI rates. Thus, the standardized infection ratio may be a preferred performance measure. The standardized infection ratio is a summary measure that is calculated by dividing the observed number of infections by the predicted number of infections. The predicted number of infections is based on infections reported to the NHSN during a baseline period and is risk adjusted based on patient care location and hospital characteristics. In addition to performing surveillance for CAUTI, hospitals may monitor compliance with process measures such as documentation of catheter insertion and removal dates and documentation of indication for catheter placement.

PREVENTION
General Strategies for Prevention

Performance of hand hygiene before and after patient care is recommended for prevention of all health care-associated infections, including CAUTI.[46] The urinary tracts of hospitalized patients and patients in long-term care facilities frequently become colonized with multidrug-resistant organisms, and patient-to-patient transmission of these organisms can occur. The use of contact precautions with gowns and gloves is recommended as part of a multifaceted strategy to prevent transmission of multidrug-resistant organisms.[47] In addition, UTI is a frequent cause of antimicrobial use in hospitalized patients.[48] Repeated antimicrobial treatment for asymptomatic bacteriuria or UTI related to long-term urinary catheterization is an important risk factor for colonization with multidrug-resistant organisms, yet much of this use of antimicrobials may be inappropriate. Reduction in use of broad spectrum antimicrobials is an important strategy to prevent development of antimicrobial resistance associated with urinary catheters. Antimicrobial stewardship programs should develop facility-specific clinical practice guidelines for the treatment of UTI.[49]

Specific Strategies for Prevention

Multiple guidelines have been developed for the prevention of CAUTI.[45,50] Key strategies for prevention of CAUTI are summarized in **Box 1**.

Limitation of Use and Early Removal of Urinary Catheters

The most effective strategy for the prevention of CAUTI is avoidance of urinary catheterization.[51] The incidence of urinary catheter placement for an inappropriate indication has been documented to be 21% to 50%.[52–54] Physician documentation of the indication for a urinary catheter has been reported to be present in less than 50% of cases.[55]

Box 1
Key strategies for prevention of catheter-associated urinary tract infection

Avoid use of indwelling urinary catheters

Place only for appropriate indications

Use alternatives to indwelling catheterization (intermittent catheterization, condom catheter, or portable bladder ultrasound scanner) when appropriate

Remove indwelling catheters early

Use nurse-based interventions

Use electronic reminders

Use proper techniques for insertion and maintenance of catheters

Adhere to sterile insertion practices

Use a closed drainage system

Avoid routine bladder irrigation

Physicians are frequently unaware of the presence of urinary catheters in their patients and this lack of awareness has been correlated with inappropriate catheter use.[56]

Indwelling urinary catheterization should be limited to certain indications (**Box 2**).[45,50] Catheters should not be inserted for convenience or for incontinence in the absence of another compelling indication. Each institution should develop written guidelines and explicit criteria for indwelling urinary catheterization based on these widely accepted indications, although modifications based on local needs may be appropriate. Regular education of medical and nursing staff regarding proper indications and supporting rationale should be undertaken. If appropriate criteria for catheter placement are not met, nursing staff should be encouraged to discuss alternatives with the ordering physician. Physician orders should be required before any catheter insertion, and institutions should implement a system for documenting the placement of catheters. Interventions for limiting urinary catheter use should be targeted at hospital locations where initial placement often occurs, such as emergency departments and operating rooms.

A number of nurse-driven interventions have demonstrated promising effectiveness in reducing the duration of catheterization. A nurse-based reminder to physicians to remove unnecessary urinary catheters in an adult ICU in a Taiwanese hospital resulted in a reduction in the incidence of CAUTI from 11.5 to 8.3 cases per 1000 catheter-days.[57] Nurse-initiated reminders to physicians of the presence of urinary catheters also decrease the number of catheter-days.[58,59] Such interventions are relatively easy to implement and may consist of either a written or electronic notice or verbal contact with the physician regarding the presence of a urinary catheter and alternative options.

The advent of electronic health records and computerized physician order entry systems allow targeted interventions both to reduce the number of catheters placed and to reduce the duration of catheterization. Cornia and colleagues[60] found that the use of a computerized reminder decreased the duration of catheterization by 3 days. In some settings, an infection prevention specialist may have the capability of working with the information technology department to integrate catheter protocols into electronic physician order entry sets.

Perioperative Management of Urinary Retention

Specific protocols for the management of perioperative urinary retention may be beneficial. Although only a limited number of prospective studies have addressed optimal postoperative bladder management strategies, indwelling urinary catheterization after

---

Box 2
Appropriate indications for placement of a urinary catheter

Accurate monitoring of urine output in a critically ill patient

Acute anatomic or functional urinary retention or obstruction

Perioperative use for selected surgical procedures

For surgical procedures of anticipated long duration

For urologic procedures

For procedures in patients with urinary incontinence

For procedures requiring intraoperative urinary monitoring or expected large volume of intravenous infusions

Urinary incontinence in patients with open perineal or sacral wounds

Improved comfort for end-of-life care, if desired

surgery has become ubiquitous in some centers. In a large cohort study, the authors demonstrated that 85% of patients admitted for major surgical procedures had perioperative indwelling catheters, and the one-half of these patients with a duration of catheterization of greater than 2 days were significantly more likely to develop UTI and less likely to be discharged to home.[61] Older surgical patients in particular are at risk for prolonged catheterization. In another study, 23% of surgical patients older than 65 years of age were discharged to skilled nursing facilities with an indwelling catheter in place and these patients were substantially more likely to be rehospitalized or die within 30 days.[62]

In a large prospective clinical trial involving orthopedic patients, the incorporation of a multifaceted protocol for perioperative catheter management resulted in a two-thirds decrease in the incidence of UTI.[63] The intervention consisted of limiting catheterization to patients who underwent surgery with a duration of more than 5 hours or who underwent total hip or knee replacement if the patient met one of several conditions. Urinary catheters were removed on postoperative day 1 after total knee arthroplasty and on postoperative day 2 after total hip arthroplasty. Although this protocol was effective at this particular hospital, each institution should develop protocols written by a local, multidisciplinary group.

Alternatives to Indwelling Urinary Catheters

Intermittent urinary catheterization may reduce the risk of UTI compared with indwelling urinary catheterization. In particular, patients with neurogenic bladder and long-term urinary catheters may benefit from intermittent catheterization. One metaanalysis demonstrated a decreased risk of asymptomatic bacteriuria and symptomatic UTI in postoperative patients after hip or knee surgery with intermittent catheterization compared with indwelling catheters (RR, 2.90), but included only 2 studies with a total of 194 patients.[64] Several studies of intermittent catheterization in postoperative patients have demonstrated increased risk of urinary retention and bladder distention.[65] Incorporating the use of a portable bladder ultrasound scanner with intermittent catheterization may attenuate this risk.[66,67]

External catheters, or condom catheters, should be considered as an alternative to indwelling catheters in appropriately selected male patients without urinary retention or bladder outlet obstruction. A randomized trial demonstrated a decrease in the composite outcome of bacteriuria, symptomatic UTI, and death in patients with condom catheters compared with patients with indwelling catheters, although the benefit was limited to those men without dementia.[68] Condom catheters may also be more comfortable than indwelling catheters.[69] More recently, external female catheters (eg, the PureWick device) have been used successfully to manage urinary incontinence.[70]

Proper Techniques for the Insertion and Maintenance of Urinary Catheters

Once a decision has been made to proceed with urinary catheterization, proper catheter insertion and maintenance are essential for prevention of CAUTI. Urinary catheters should be inserted using sterile equipment and aseptic technique by a trained health care practitioner.[45,50] Cleaning of the meatal area should be undertaken before catheter insertion, but there is currently no consensus regarding the use of sterile water compared with the use of an antiseptic preparation. A randomized study comparing sterile water with 0.1% chlorhexidine for cleaning of the meatal area before insertion demonstrated no difference in the development of bacteriuria.[71] Ongoing catheter maintenance with daily meatal cleaning using an antiseptic has also not shown a clear benefit and it may actually increase rates of bacteriuria compared with routine care with soap and water.[72] A single-use packet of sterile lubricant jelly should be used for insertion to reduce urethral trauma, but it does not need to possess antiseptic properties.[50] Urinary catheters should not be routinely exchanged, except for mechanical reasons, because any reduction in the rate of bacteriuria with routine changing is generally only transient.[73]

The use of closed urinary catheter systems with sealed catheter–tubing junctions reduces the risk of CAUTI.[45,50] Breaches of the closed system should be avoided and urine should be sampled only from a port after cleaning with an antiseptic solution or from the drainage bag using sterile technique if a large sample is required. Breach of the closed system to instill antibiotics is associated with increased rates of infection and irrigation of the bladder with antibiotics can cause the organisms colonizing the catheter biofilm to flow into the bladder.[74]

Antiinfective Catheters

Use of antiseptic and antibiotic-impregnated urinary catheters may have an impact on the rates of catheter-associated bacteriuria. Antiseptic catheters currently available are coated with silver alloy. Earlier catheters coated with silver oxide lacked efficacy compared with silver alloy–coated catheters and are no longer available. Other antibiotic-impregnated catheters have used various types of antibiotics, including nitrofurazone, minocycline, and rifampin.

In a large metaanalysis, use of silver alloy–coated catheters significantly reduced the incidence of asymptomatic bacteriuria (RR, 0.54) among adult patients catheterized for less than 7 days compared with use of latex catheters.[75] Among patients catheterized for more than 7 days, a decrease in asymptomatic bacteriuria was less pronounced (RR, 0.64). In the same metaanalysis, antibiotic-impregnated catheters were compared with standard catheters and were found to decrease the rate of asymptomatic bacteriuria (RR, 0.52) for duration of catheterization less than 7 days, but demonstrated no benefit for duration of catheterization of more than 7 days. Another metaanalysis demonstrated similar reductions in asymptomatic bacteriuria in patients with short-term catheterization.[76] There are few trials assessing antiseptic- and antibiotic-coated catheters in patients with long-term urinary catheterization, and no conclusions can be drawn regarding such patients.[77]

The use of antiinfective urinary catheters seems to be 1 option to decrease the incidence of bacteriuria in patients with short-term urinary catheterization (for <7 days), but the effect on the more important outcomes of symptomatic CAUTI and urinary catheter-associated bloodstream infection are not clear from the current literature. The current consensus is that antiinfective urinary catheters should not be used routinely to prevent CAUTI.[45]

Implementation, Bladder Bundles, and Collaboratives

Strategies to prevent CAUTI have not been implemented uniformly at US hospitals. Therefore, more recent research on CAUTI prevention has focused on implementation of strategies that are known to be effective in reducing CAUTI rates. A 2013 survey of select US hospitals found that only 39% routinely monitored urinary catheter duration and/or discontinuation, 39% performed bladder ultrasound examinations, and 23% had catheter reminders or stop orders and/or nurse-initiated discontinuation.[78]

To improve compliance with CAUTI prevention measures, many hospitals have participated in collaboratives. For example, the Michigan Hospital Association Keystone Center launched a statewide initiative in 2007 to decrease health care-associated infections, including CAUTI.[79] As a part of this initiative, participating hospitals adopted a bladder bundle, that is, a set of preventive practices consisting of nurse-initiated urinary catheter discontinuation, urinary catheter reminders and removal prompts, alternatives to indwelling catheterization, portable bladder ultrasound examinations, and insertion care and maintenance. The key components of the collaborative model were engagement of hospital leadership and health care providers, education, execution, and evaluation. In the same 2013 survey described, Michigan hospitals were found to have higher rates of compliance with preventive measures after the implementation of the bladder bundle, as well as a 25% decrease in CAUTI rates statewide, compared with a 6% decrease nationally.[78]

SUMMARY

CAUTIs are common, costly, and cause significant patient morbidity. Despite studies showing benefit of interventions for prevention of CAUTI, adoption of these practices has not occurred consistently in many health care facilities in the United States. The duration of urinary catheterization is the predominant risk for CAUTI; preventive measures directed at limiting placement and early removal of urinary catheters have a significant impact on decreasing CAUTI. Intervention bundles, collaboratives, and support from hospital leadership are powerful tools for implementing preventive measures for health care-associated infections, including CAUTI.

REFERENCES

1. Magill S, Edwards J, Bamberg W, et al. Multistate point-prevalence survey of health care-associated infections. N Engl J Med 2014;370(13):1198–208.
2. Chenoweth C, Saint S. Urinary tract infections. Infect Dis Clin North Am 2016;30: 869–85.
3. Burton D, Edwards J, Srinivasan A, et al. Trends in catheter-associated urinary tract infection in adult intensive care units-United States, 1990-2007. Infect Control Hosp Epidemiol 2011;32:748–56.
4. Mitchell B, Ferguson J, Anderson M, et al. Length of stay and mortality associated with healthcare-associated urinary tract infections: a multi-state model. J Hosp Infect 2016;93(1):92–9.
5. Zimlichman E, Henderson D, Tamir O, et al. Health care-associated infections: a meta-analysis of costs and financial impact on the US care system. JAMA Intern Med 2013;173(22):2039–46.
6. Umsheid C, Mitchell M, Doshi J, et al. Estimating the proportion of healthcare-associated infections that are reasonably preventable and the related mortality and costs. Infect Control Hosp Epidemiol 2011;32(2):101–14.
7. Saint S, Meddings JA, Calfee D, et al. Catheter-associated urinary tract infection and the Medicare rule changes. Ann Intern Med 2009;150(12):877–84.
8. Dudeck M, Edwards J, Allen-Bridson K, et al. National Healthcare Safety Network (NHSN) report, data summary for 2013, device associated module. Am J Infect Control 2015;43(3):206–21.
9. Metersky M, Eldridge N, Wang Y, et al. National trends in the frequency of bladder catheterization and physician-diagnoses catheter-associated urinary tract infections: results from the Medicare Patient Safety Monitoring System. Am J Infect Control 2017;45(8):901–4.
10. Saint S, Greene T, Krein S, et al. A program to prevent catheter-associated urinary tract infection in acute care. N Engl J Med 2016;374(22):2111–9.
11. Patrick S, Kawai A, Kleinman K, et al. Health care-associated infections among critically ill children in the US, 2007-2012. Pediatrics 2014;134(4):705–12.

12. Lewis S, Knelson L, Moehring R, et al. Comparison of non-intensive care unit (ICU) versus ICU rates of catheter-associated infections in community hospitals. Infect Control Hosp Epidemiol 2013;34(7):744–7.

13. Rosenthal V, Al-Abdeli H, El-Kholy A, et al. International nosocomial infection control consortium report, data summary of 50 countries for 2010-2015: device-associated module. Am J Infect Control 2016;44:1495–504.

14. Weiner L, Fridkin S, Aponte-Torres Z, et al. Vital signs: preventing antibiotic-resistant infections in hospitals- United States, 2014. MMWR Morb Mortal Wkly Rep 2016;65(9):235–41.

15. Weiner L, Webb A, Limbago B, et al. Antimicrobial-resistant pathogens associated with healthcare-associated infections: summary of the data reported to the National Healthcare Safety Network at the centers for disease control and prevention, 2011-2014. Infect Control Hosp Epidemiol 2016;37(11):1288–301.

16. Lake J, Weiner L, Milstone A, et al. Pathogen distribution and antimicrobial resistance among pediatric healthcare-associated infections reported to the National Healthcare Safety Network, 2011-2014. Infect Control Hosp Epidemiol 2018; 39(1):1–11.

17. Chenoweth C, Saint S. Preventing catheter-associated urinary tract infections in the intensive care unit. Crit Care Clin 2013;29:19–32.

18. Chang R, Green MT, Chenoweth CE, et al. Epidemiology of hospital-acquired urinary tract-related bloodstream infection at a university hospital. Infect Control Hosp Epidemiol 2011;32(11):1127–9.

19. Greene MT, Chang R, Kuhn L, et al. Predictors of hospital-acquired urinary tract-related bloodstream infection. Infect Control Hosp Epidemiol 2012;33(10): 1001–7.

20. Kizilbash Q, Petersen N, Chen G, et al. Bacteremia and mortality with urinary catheter-associated bacteriuria. Infect Control Hosp Epidemiol 2013;34(11): 1153–9.

21. Krieger JN, Kaiser DL, Wenzel RP. Urinary tract etiology of bloodstream infections in hospitalized patients. J Infect Dis 1983;148(1):57–62.

22. Saint S, Kaufman SR, Rogers MA, et al. Risk factors for nosocomial urinary tract-related bacteremia: a case-control study. Am J Infect Control 2006;34(7):401–7.

23. Tambyah PA, Halvorson KT, Maki DG. A prospective study of pathogenesis of catheter-associated urinary tract infections. Mayo Clin Proc 1999;74:131–6.

24. Saint S, Chenoweth CE. Biofilms and catheter-associated urinary tract infections. Infect Dis Clin North Am 2003;17:411–32.

25. Nicolle L. Catheter associated urinary tract infection. Antimicrob Resist Infect Control 2014;3:23.

26. Bossa L, Kline K, McDougald D, et al. Urinary catheter-associated microbiota change in accordance with treatment and infection status. PLoS One 2017; 12(6):e0177633.

27. Walker J, Flores-Mireles A, Pinkner C, et al. Catheterization alters bladder ecology to potentiate Staphylococcus aureus infection of the urinary tract. Proc Natl Acad Sci U S A 2017;114(14):E8721–30.

28. Wang J, Foxman B, Mody L, et al. Network of microbial and antibiotic interactions drive colonization and infection with multidrug-resistant organisms. Proc Natl Acad Sci U S A 2017;114(39):10467–72.

29. Tambyah PA, Maki DG. Catheter-associated urinary tract infection is rarely symptomatic: a prospective study of 1,497 catheterized patients. Arch Intern Med 2000;160(5):678–82.

30. Tambyah PA, Maki DG. The relationship between pyuria and infection in patients with indwelling urinary catheters: a prospective study of 761 patients. Arch Intern Med 2000;160(5):673–7.

31. Jones K, Sibai J, Battjes R, et al. How and why nurses collect urine cultures on catheterized patients: a survey of 5 hospitals. Am J Infect Control 2016;44(2): 173–6.

32. LaRocca M, Franek J, Leibach E, et al. Effectiveness of preanalytic practices on contamination and diagnostic accuracy of urine cultures: a laboratory medicine best practices systematic review and meta-analysis. Clin Microbiol Rev 2016; 29(1):105–47.

33. Hartley S, Valley S, Kuhn L, et al. Inappropriate testing for urinary tract infection in hospitalized patients: an opportunity of improvement. Infect Control Hosp Epidemiol 2013;34(11):1204–7.

34. Horstman M, Spiegelman A, Naik A, et al. National patterns of urine testing during inpatient admission. Clin Infect Dis 2017;65(7):1199–205.

35. Tedja R, Wentink J, O'Horo J, et al. Catheter-associated urinary tract infections in intensive care unit patients. Infect Control Hosp Epidemiol 2015;36(11):1330–4.

36. Grein J, Kahn K, Eells S, et al. Treatment of positive urine cultures in hospitalized adults: a survey of prevalence and risk factors in 3 medical centers. Infect Control Hosp Epidemiol 2016;37(3):319–26.

37. Hartley S, Valley S, Kuhn L, et al. Overtreatment of asymptomatic bacteriuria: identifying targets for improvement. Infect Control Hosp Epidemiol 2015;36(4): 470–3.

38. Trautner B, Petersen N, Hysong S, et al. Overtreatment of asymptomatic bacteriuria, identifying barriers to evidence-based care. Am J Infect Control 2014;42(6): 653–8.

39. Nicolle L, Bradley S, Colgan R, et al. Infectious Diseases Society of America guidelines for the diagnosis and treatment of asymptomatic bacteriuria in adults. Clin Infect Dis 2005;40:643–54.

40. Hartley S, Kuhn L, Valley S, et al. Evaluating a hospitalist-based intervention to decrease unnecessary antimicrobial use in patients with asymptomatic bacteriuria. Infect Control Hosp Epidemiol 2016;37(9):1044–51.

41. Trautner B, Grigoryan L, Petersen N, et al. Effectiveness of an antimicrobial stewardship approach for urinary catheter-associated asymptomatic bacteriuria. JAMA Intern Med 2015;175(7):1120–7.

42. Centers for Disease Control and Prevention. Urinary tract infection (catheter-associated urinary tract infection [CAUTI] and non-catheter associated urinary tract infection [UTI]) and other urinary tract system (USI) events. Available at: https://www.cdc.gov/nhsn/pdfs/pscmanual/7psccauticurrent.pdf. Accessed February 1, 2018.

43. Centers for Disease Control and Prevention. Operational guidance for acute care hospitals to report catheter-associated urinary tract infection (CAUTI) data to CDC's NHSN for the purpose of fulfilling CMS's hospital Inpatient Quality Reporting (IQR) requirements. Available at: https://www.cdc.gov/nhsn/pdfs/cms/Final-ACH-CAUTI-Guidance_2015.pdf. Accessed February 1, 2018.

44. Centers for Medicare and Medicaid Services (CMS). Hospital compare. Available at: https://www.medicare.gov/hospitalcompare/search.html. Accessed February 1, 2018.

45. Lo E, Nicolle LE, Coffin SE, et al. Strategies to prevent catheter-associated urinary tract infection in acute care hospitals: 2014 update. Infect Control Hosp Epidemiol 2014;35(S2):S32–47.

46. Boyce JM, Pittet D. Guideline for hand hygiene in healthcare settings: recommendations of the Healthcare Infection Control Practices Advisory Committee and the HICPAC/SHEA/APIC/IDSA Hand Hygiene Task Force. Society for Healthcare Epidemiology of America/Association for Professionals in Infection Control/Infectious Diseases Society of America. MMWR Recomm Rep 2002;51(RR-16):1–45.

47. Siegel JD, Rhinehart E, Jackson M, et al. 2007 Guideline for isolation precautions: preventing transmission of infectious agents in health care settings. Am J Infect Control 2007;35(10 Suppl 2):S65–164.

48. Gandhi T, Flanders SA, Markovitz E, et al. Importance of urinary tract infection to antibiotic use among hospitalized patients. Infect Control Hosp Epidemiol 2009; 30(2):193–5.

49. Barlam TF, Cosgrove SE, Abbo LM, et al. Implementing an antibiotic stewardship program: guidelines by the Infectious Diseases Society of America and the Society for Healthcare Epidemiology of America. Clin Infect Dis 2016;62(10):e51–77.

50. Gould CV, Umscheid CA, Agarwal RK, et al. Guideline for prevention of catheter-associated urinary tract infections 2009. Available at: https://www.cdc.gov/infectioncontrol/pdf/guidelines/cauti-guidelines.pdf. Accessed February 1, 2018.

51. Nicolle LE. The prevention of hospital-acquired urinary tract infection. Clin Infect Dis 2008;46(2):251–3.

52. Gardam MA, Amihod B, Orenstein P, et al. Overutilization of indwelling urinary catheters and the development of nosocomial urinary tract infections. Clin Perform Qual Health Care 1998;6(3):99–102.

53. Jain P, Parada JP, David A, et al. Overuse of the indwelling urinary tract catheter in hospitalized medical patients. Arch Intern Med 1995;155(13):1425–9.

54. Munasinghe RL, Yazdani H, Siddique M, et al. Appropriateness of use of indwelling urinary catheters in patients admitted to the medical service. Infect Control Hosp Epidemiol 2001;22(10):647–9.

55. Conybeare A, Pathak S, Imam I. The quality of hospital records of urethral catheterisation. Ann R Coll Surg Engl 2002;84(2):109–10.

56. Saint C, Wiooo J, Amory JK, et al. Are physicians aware of which of their patients have indwelling catheters? Am J Med 2000;109:476–80.

57. Huang WC, Wann SR, Lin SL, et al. Catheter-associated urinary tract infections in intensive care units can be reduced by prompting physicians to remove unnecessary catheters. Infect Control Hosp Epidemiol 2004;25(11):974–8.

58. Fakih MG, Dueweke C, Meisner S, et al. Effect of nurse-led multidisciplinary rounds on reducing the unnecessary use of urinary catheterization in hospitalized patients. Infect Control Hosp Epidemiol 2008;29(9):815–9.

59. Saint S, Kaufman SR, Thompson M, et al. A reminder reduces urinary catheterization in hospitalized patients. Jt Comm J Qual Patient Saf 2005;31(8):455–62.

60. Cornia PB, Amory JK, Fraser S, et al. Computer-based order entry decreases duration of indwelling urinary catheterization in hospitalized patients. Am J Med 2003;114(5):404–7.

61. Wald HL, Ma A, Bratzler DW, et al. Indwelling urinary catheter use in the postoperative period: analysis of the national surgical infection prevention project data. Arch Surg 2008;143(6):551–7.

62. Wald HL, Epstein AM, Radcliff TA, et al. Extended use of urinary catheters in older surgical patients: a patient safety problem? Infect Control Hosp Epidemiol 2008; 29(2):116–24.

63. Stephan F, Sax H, Wachsmuth M, et al. Reduction of urinary tract infection and antibiotic use after surgery: a controlled, prospective, before-after intervention study. Clin Infect Dis 2006;42(11):1544–51.

64. Niel-Weise BS, van den Broek PJ. Urinary catheter policies for short-term bladder drainage in adults. Cochrane Database Syst Rev 2005;(3):CD004203.
65. Oishi CS, Williams VJ, Hanson PB, et al. Perioperative bladder management after primary total hip arthroplasty. J Arthroplasty 1995;10(6):732–6.
66. Moore DA, Edwards K. Using a portable bladder scan to reduce the incidence of nosocomial urinary tract infections. Medsurg Nurs 1997;6(1):39–43.
67. Stevens E. Bladder ultrasound: avoiding unnecessary catheterizations. Medsurg Nurs 2005;14(4):249–53.
68. Saint S, Kaufman SR, Rogers MA, et al. Condom versus indwelling urinary catheters: a randomized trial. J Am Geriatr Soc 2006;54(7):1055–61.
69. Saint S, Lipsky BA, Baker PD, et al. Urinary catheters: what type do men and their nurses prefer? J Am Geriatr Soc 1999;47(12):1453–7.
70. Beeston T, Davis C. Urinary management with an external female collection device. J Wound Ostomy Continence Nurs 2018;45(2):187–9.
71. Webster J, Hood RH, Burridge CA, et al. Water or antiseptic for periurethral cleaning before urinary catheterization: a randomized controlled trial. Am J Infect Control 2001;29(6):389–94.
72. Burke JP, Garibaldi RA, Britt MR, et al. Prevention of catheter-associated urinary tract infections. Efficacy of daily meatal care regimens. Am J Med 1981;70(3):655–8.
73. Tenney JH, Warren JW. Bacteriuria in women with long-term catheters: paired comparison of indwelling and replacement catheters. J Infect Dis 1988;157(1):199–202.
74. Warren JW, Platt R, Thomas RJ, et al. Antibiotic irrigation and catheter-associated urinary-tract infections. N Engl J Med 1978;299(11):570–3.
75. Saint S, Elmore J, Sullivan S, et al. The efficacy of silver alloy-coated urinary catheters in preventing urinary tract infection: a meta-analysis. Am J Med 1998;105:236–41.
76. Johnson JR, Kuskowski MA, Wilt TJ. Systematic review: antimicrobial urinary catheters to prevent catheter-associated urinary tract infection in hospitalized patients. Ann Intern Med 2006;144(2):116–26.
77. Jahn P, Preuss M, Kernig A, et al. Types of indwelling urinary catheters for long-term bladder drainage in adults. Cochrane Database Syst Rev 2007;(3):CD004997.
78. Saint S, Greene MT, Kowalski CP, et al. Preventing catheter-associated urinary tract infection in the United States: a national comparative study. JAMA Intern Med 2013;173(10):874–9.
79. Saint S, Olmsted RN, Fakih MG, et al. Translating healthcare-associated urinary tract infection prevention research into practice via the bladder bundle. Jt Comm J Qual Patient Saf 2009;35(9):449–55.

New Developments in the Prevention of Gastrointestinal Scope-Related Infections

Jonathan D. Grein, MD[a], Rekha K. Murthy, MD, FRCPC[a,b,*]

KEYWORDS

- Gastrointestinal endoscopy • Duodenoscopes • High level disinfection
- Endoscopic retrograde cholangiopancreatography (ERCP)
- Carbapenem-resistant *Enterobacteriaceae*

KEY POINTS

- Gastrointestinal endoscopy has been associated with more health care-associated outbreaks than any other medical device.
- Recent outbreaks related to duodenoscopes have occurred at health care institutions despite following current guidelines.
- Prevention of infection after gastrointestinal endoscopy requires strict adherence to current guidelines for cleaning and disinfection.
- Research is needed on optimal methods of cleaning and disinfection/sterilization of duodenoscopes in the setting of new endoscope design features, increase in multidrug resistance, and presence of biofilms.

INTRODUCTION

Endoscopes are medical devices used for used for diagnostic and therapeutic procedures involving the gastrointestinal (GI) tract. The minimally invasive nature of GI endoscopy makes it a preferred procedure in diagnostics and surgery. Modern endoscopy techniques have revolutionized the examination and treatment of the upper GI tract and colon. The prevalence and complexity of these procedures has increased, as has their capability of providing a greater variety of procedures and sometimes providing important alternatives to spare more invasive surgical procedures.

Disclosure Statement: The authors have no disclosures relevant to the content of this article.
[a] Department of Hospital Epidemiology, Division of Infectious Diseases, Cedars-Sinai Medical Center, 8635 W 3rd Street, Suite 1150W, Los Angeles, CA, USA; [b] Department of Medical Affairs, Cedars-Sinai Medical Center, 8700 Beverly Boulevard, Suite 2211, Los Angeles, CA 90048, USA
* Corresponding author. Department of Medical Affairs, Cedars-Sinai Medical Center, 8700 Beverly Boulevard, Suite 2211, Los Angeles, CA 90048.
E-mail address: Rekha.Murthy@cshs.org

Infect Dis Clin N Am 32 (2018) 899–913
https://doi.org/10.1016/j.idc.2018.06.008
0891-5520/18/© 2018 Elsevier Inc. All rights reserved.

id.theclinics.com

About 20 million GI endoscopic procedures are performed annually in the United States.[1] Infectious complications of GI endoscopy are well-described and their risk varies based on the procedure and underlying patient risk factors; they can be divided into those involving translocation of the patients own flora (endogenous) or those involving transmission of organisms to patients via contaminated equipment (exogenous).

Recent reports of exogenous infections with multidrug-resistant (MDR) bacteria transmitted via contaminated endoscopic retrograde cholangiopancreatography (ERCP) duodenoscopes have underscored the critical role of cleaning and reprocessing of reusable endoscopic equipment. Increasing complexity in newer duodenoscope design has contributed to these challenges.[2] Revisions to endoscope reprocessing guidelines, as well as duodenoscope design and manufacturer reprocessing instructions, have been implemented recently to mitigate ongoing risks of exogenous infection from contaminated endoscopes.[3]

The focus of this review is to provide an overview of recent developments and the current understanding of the key contributing factors related to GI endoscope-related infections, as well as of current approaches to identify and prevent these complications.

BACKGROUND

GI endoscopy is one of the most widely performed medical procedures in the world.[1] Endoscopic GI procedures can be divided into those involving the upper or lower GI tract and can be performed for diagnostic or therapeutic purposes (or both). Lower endoscopy (colonoscopy, sigmoidoscopy) provides for visualization from the rectum to distal ileum and has many indications, including colorectal cancer screening and diagnosis, and management of lower GI bleeding. Upper endoscopy (esophagogastroduodenoscopy) allows visualization from the oropharynx to the proximal duodenum, and is commonly performed for several indications, including upper GI bleeding (ulcer or variceal in origin), esophageal reflux, dysphagia, management of esophageal strictures, and malignancy screening. ERCP allows for detailed evaluation of the biliary system (through the ampulla of Vater) and requires a side-viewing duodenoscope.[4,5]

Flexible endoscopes have complex internal structures with multiple internal channels that allow for manipulation of the tip, visualization (fiberoptic light source and imaging cables), deployment of air and water, and retrieval of biopsy material.[6] Flushing and drying of these channels is a critical component of reprocessing; multiple outbreaks involving *Pseudomonas*, *Serratia*, and *Mycobacteria* have been linked with inadequate drying.[6]

Side-viewing endoscopes (duodenoscopes used for ERCP) have an additional unique feature, a cantilevered elevator mechanism at the distal tip controlled by an elevator wire (via a dedicated channel).[2,5] This design is challenging to clean and disinfect and has been proposed as a contributing factor to recent outbreaks associated with duodenoscopes.

Peery and colleagues[1] reported increasing trends, between 2000 and 2009, in both upper and lower GI endoscopy of 54% and 17%, respectively. There were an estimated 6.9 million upper, 11.5 million lower, and 228,000 biliary endoscopies performed in the United States in 2009 based on Thompson Reuters MarketScan commercial, Medicare, and Medicaid databases. An estimated 668,000 ERCPs were performed in the United States in 2014, representing a 14% increase from 2010.[7] ERCP is increasingly being used for therapeutic indications rather than for conventional diagnostic purposes.[8]

INFECTIONS AFTER GASTROINTESTINAL ENDOSCOPY
Endogenous Infections

Endogenous infections are attributed to breaches in the mucosal barrier during the procedure and secondary infection with the patient's own bacterial flora. The risk of endogenous infection is highly variable and depends the nature of the procedure as well as underlying patient risk factors. Infections may range from transient bacteremia to sepsis, peritonitis, abscess, or endocarditis. Flexible sigmoidoscopy is associated with low rates of transient bacteremia ($\leq$1%), whereas bacteremia rates may be higher for colonoscopy (0%–25%) or diagnostic upper endoscopy (<8%).[6] Therapeutic upper endoscopic procedures (variceal ligation, sclerotherapy, or esophageal dilation) are associated with higher rates of bacteremia ($\leq$54%).[6,9]

Severe infectious complications occur after ERCP in 2% to 4% of patients and may include bacteremia, ascending cholangitis, cholecystitis, liver abscess, and necrotizing pancreatitis.[4] Infection risk is higher when biliary obstruction is present versus absent and higher when an obstruction is malignant versus benign. Sepsis after ERCP may have a mortality rate as high as 29%.[6]

The spectrum of flora involved reflect the anatomic location manipulated; upper endoscopic procedures often involve coagulase-negative *Staphylococcus* and *Streptococcus*, whereas lower endoscopic procedures and ERCP often involve *Enterobacteriaceae*, enterococci, and alpha-hemolytic *Streptococcus*.[10] The risk of MDR *Enterobacteriaceae* infection, such as extended-spectrum beta-lactamase–producing organisms or carbapenem-resistant *Enterobacteriaceae* (CRE), continue to increase, although data on MDR infections attributed to endoscopy are not available. In South Korea, rates of bacteremic biliary tract infection with an organism resistant to third-generation cephalosporins increased from 25% in 2000 to 2004 to 48% in 2005 to 2009; rates of extended-spectrum beta-lactamase–producing *Escherichia coli* and *Klebsiella* increased from 2% to 44% during the same period.[11] In the United States, the prevalence of extended-spectrum beta-lactamase–producing *Klebsiella pneumoniae* in intraabdominal cultures increased from 3.2% in 2005 to 13.1% in 2010, and the overall proportion of *Enterobacteriaceae* that are CRE increased from 1.2% in 2001 to 4.2% in 2011.[12,13]

Exogenous Infections

Contaminated endoscopes are the most common cause of device related nosocomial outbreaks in the United States.[6,14] The investigation of recent outbreaks have yielded information about the factors that may contribute to risk of infection. Exogenous infections are typically a result of microorganisms introduced by the endoscope or its accessory equipment that can be transmitted from patients who have previously undergone endoscopy with the same device. The prevalence of infections resulting from transmission of pathogens from endoscopic procedures is undoubtedly underestimated owing to their low frequency, lack of validated surveillance methods, and potential for undetected asymptomatic or subclinical symptoms or signs. Data from 63 published reports include more than 500 episodes of microbial transmission, with a recent increase between 2010 to 2015 involving more than 170 patients related to transmission of MDR gram-negative bacteria.[10] Exogenous infections are preventable with strict adherence to accepted reprocessing guidelines.

Pseudomonas aeruginosa has been the most common bacterial pathogens reported with GI endoscopy since introduction of multisociety guidelines on high-level disinfection (HLD), particularly during ERCP. *P aeruginosa*, a gram-negative pathogen found in the health care environment, has a predilection for producing biofilm, particularly in moist environments (such as wet endoscope channels and plumbing), which are very difficult to remove.[10,15] The most common factors associated with microbial transmission during GI endoscopy involve inadequate cleaning, disinfection, and drying procedures; the use of contaminated automated endoscope reprocessors (AERs), and flaws in instrument design or use of damaged endoscopes.

Only 1 report of *C difficile* transmission has been published. Viral transmission (hepatitis B and C) has also been described, although much less frequently. Although theoretically possible, transmission of human immunodeficiency virus, enterovirus, or prions (Creutzfeldt-Jacob disease) has not been observed to date.[6]

Multidrug-Resistant Organisms

Recent outbreaks associated with MDR organisms (MDRO) have drawn attention not only to the importance of their detection and prevention, but also to the potential contribution of design changes in newer devices to risk of infection from potentially inadequate current cleaning protocols. The severity of illness and limited treatment options of MDRO infections has contributed to the urgency of collaboration between health care facilities, device manufacturers, and regulatory agencies to address the risks of GI endoscopy–related exogenous infection.

The emergence of MDRO in the United States, particularly that of CRE and gram negatives, has been designated an urgent public health threat by the Centers for Disease Control and Prevention (CDC).[16] Infections associated with CRE and other MDRO are associated with high mortality rates owing to severity of illness and, because these organisms are resistant to almost all classes of antimicrobial agents, limiting treatment options.[17] Some CRE possess a beta-lactamase (eg, AmpC or extended spectrum beta-lactamase) which, when combined with porin mutations, can render an organism nonsusceptible to carbapenems. In addition, some CRE possess carbapenemases that directly break down carbapenems and may reside on mobile plasmids that can be transmitted to other bacteria.

Although not clearly established, transmission of CRE and other MDRO may be associated with a higher risk of infection compared with usual enteric organisms because standard antimicrobial prophylaxis is not effective for CRE and because MDR *Klebsiella* and other bacteria may be more adept at generating biofilms that may hinder routine cleaning of endoscopes.[18] For these reasons, the detection of CRE and other MDRO may serve as an early indicator for identifying ineffective reprocessing of duodenoscopes.[19]

OUTBREAKS ASSOCIATED WITH GASTROINTESTINAL ENDOSCOPES

Historically, infectious complications of GI endoscopy procedures were considered rare and estimated to occur once every 1.8 million procedures, although reporting bias and lack of comprehensive surveillance likely contribute to a significant underestimate of the true burden.[20] Nonetheless, between 1966 and 2005, 70 endoscope-related outbreaks were reported and more than 90% were considered preventable through improved quality control systems.[21] Until recently, lapses in endoscope reprocessing were identified in nearly all outbreaks. Water-associated pathogens, including *P aeruginosa* and *Mycobacteria spp*, have been the most frequently organism involved, likely related to their propensity for biofilm formation and tolerance to disinfectants.[6] Additionally, *Salmonella spp* are resistant to less potent disinfectant solutions and were frequently associated with outbreaks until the use of more potent disinfectants was instituted.[6,22] More recently, MDR *Enterobacteriaceae* have become frequently associated with outbreaks, where lapses in nearly every step of endoscope reprocessing were implicated, reflecting the low margin of safety in HLD of semicritical devices.[15] Inadequate cleaning and bioburden removal, inadequate use or tolerance to disinfectants, contaminated AERs, contaminated flushing of channels, inadequate drying, and persistence of biofilm formation have all contributed to pathogen transmission.[6]

Although AERs can improve the standardization of reprocessing and are the preferred approach for HLD, defective or contaminated AERs have also contributed to multiple outbreaks.[23,24] Recently, AERs have been implicated in transmission of MDRO transmission from duodenoscopes. In November 2015, the US Food and Drug Administration (FDA) recalled a Custom Ultrasonic AER, citing the company for failing to validate adequate endoscope disinfection. In August 2016, the FDA revised its recall to apply only to duodenoscopes given lack of evidence that the AER was associated with transmission with nonduodenoscope endoscopes.[25]

Biofilm formation on endoscopes plays an important role in facilitating transmission. Bacteria often implicated in endoscope outbreaks, such as *Pseudomonas* and atypical *Mycobacteria*, can readily develop biofilm in the presence of bioburden or moisture, which can be resistant to cleaning and disinfectants.[10] Additionally, routine wear after repeated use may facilitate biofilm formation, although no current standards exist to routinely replace endoscopes after repeated use.[26]

Until recent outbreaks, HLD done in accordance with previously published multisociety guidelines and manufacturers' recommendations were considered adequate to safeguard patients from risk of infection transmission.[27] Recent outbreaks associated with ERCP procedures have occurred despite apparently appropriate cleaning and HLD. The details of these episodes highlight the challenges with consistent clearance of all organisms from the exposed, complex, moving parts and operating channels of duodenoscopes and the potential role of biofilms in hindering adequate reprocessing.[2,28] Between 2012 and early 2015, at least 35 different instances of antibiotic-resistant infections affecting at least 250 patients worldwide have been linked to closed-channel duodenoscope models made by all 3 major manufacturers (Olympus, Pentax, and Fujifilm).[5] **Table 1** provides a summary of the outbreaks, the number of patients affected, and the type of duodenoscope; these outbreaks have been linked to MDRO that are associated with high mortality rates. More than 1000 potentially exposed patients have been advised to undergo screening cultures and at least 100 patients are believed to harbor silent carriage of the outbreak-associated organisms.[3]

These outbreaks have led the FDA and the CDC to reappraise the risks associated with duodenoscopes. The FDA's final report determined that the complex design of duodenoscopes may impede effective reprocessing and that duodenoscope-related outbreaks are occurring despite adherence to manufacturers' instructions for use and professional guidelines.[28] Transmission is attributed to persistent contamination at the elevator region and/or the elevator cable and has occurred with instrument designs from all major duodenoscope manufacturers.

ENDOSCOPE REPROCESSING

The Spaulding classification is the accepted approach to categorizing medical devices by infection risk and determining the type of disinfection required for reprocessing.[29] Devices are considered noncritical if they only contact intact skin (ie, stethoscopes), semicritical if they contact mucosa (ie, endoscopes), or critical if they are used within sterile tissue (ie, surgical instruments). Low-level disinfection, such as wiping a surface with a disinfectant wipe, is acceptable between use of noncritical devices. Semicritical devices require HLD, which use disinfectants

Table 1
Summary of MDR outbreaks linked to duodenoscopes, 2010-2015

Hospital (Outbreak Pathogen, Where Available)	Estimated No. of Patients Infected	Approximate Date of Infections	Duodenoscope Manufacturer
Erasmus Medical Center, Rotterdam, the Netherlands (VIM-2-positive *Pseudomonas aeruginosa*)[46]	30	January 2012	Olympus
Clinique De Bercy, Charenton-le-Pont, France	3	October 2012	Olympus
University of Pittsburgh Medical Center Presbyterian Hospital, Pittsburgh, PA (CRKP)[47]	135	November 2012	Olympus
New York-Presbyterian/Weill Cornell Medical Center, New York, NY	15	December 2012	Olympus
UMass Memorial Medical Center, Worchester, MA	20	Dec-12	Olympus
Carolinas Medical Center, Charlotte, NC (CRE)	1	2013	Olympus
Thomas Jefferson University Hospital, Philadelphia, PA (CRE)	8	January 2013	Olympus
Charite-Universitatsmedizin, Berlin, Germany (CRKP)[48]	5	February 2013	Olympus
Advocate Lutheran General Hospital, Park Ridge, IL (NDM-1 E. coli)	32	March 2013	Pentax
Froedtert Hospital, Milwaukee, WI (NDM-1 *Escherichia coli*)[49]	5	May 2013	Olympus
Virginia Mason Hospital and Medical Center, Seattle, WA (Hyper-ampC *E coli*)[50]	32	Spring/summer 2013	Olympus
Clinique De Bercy, Charenton-Le-Pont, France	2	November 2013	Olympus
Hartford Hospital, Hartford, CT (MDR-*E coli*)	12	January 2014	Olympus
Massachusetts General Hospital, Boston, MA	7	Before Spring 2014	Pentax
Advocate Good Samaritan Hospital, Downers Grove, IL	3	May 2014	Fujifilm
Evangelisches Waldkrankenhaus, Spandau, Berlin, Germany	4	May 2014	Olympus
Boca Raton Regional Hospital, Boca Raton, FL	96	August 2014	Olympus
Cedars-Sinai Medical Center, Los Angeles, CA (CRKP)[51]	4	August 2014	Olympus
UCLA Medical Center, Los Angeles, CA (CRKP OXA 32)[52]	7	October 2014	Olympus
Carolinas Medical Center, Charlotte, NC	18	2015	Olympus
MGH Gastroenterology Associates, Boston, MA	5	January 2015	Pentax
Massachusetts General Hospital, Boston, MA	3	January 2015	Pentax

(continued on next page)

Table 1 (continued)			
Hospital (Outbreak Pathogen, Where Available)	Estimated No. of Patients Infected	Approximate Date of Infections	Duodenoscope Manufacturer
Universitair Medisch Centrum, Utrecht, the Netherlands	8	January 2015	Olympus
Allegheny General Hospital, Pittsburgh, PA	1	February 2015	Olympus
Fox Chase Cancer Center, Philadelphia, PA	3	April 2015	Fujifilm

Abbreviations: CRE, carbapenem-resistant *Enterobacteriaceae*; CRKP, carbapenem-resistant *Klebsiella pneumoniae*; MDR, multidrug resistant.
Data from Rubin ZA, Murthy RK. Outbreaks associated with duodenoscopes: new challenges and controversies. Curr Opin Infect Dis 2016;29:407–14; and *Adapted from* US Senate. Senate health, education, labor and pensions committee & minority staff report: preventable tragedies: super-bugs and how ineffective monitoring of medical device safety fails patients. Patty Murray, Ranking Member Jan 13, 2016. Available at: https://www.help.senate.gov/imo/media/doc/Duodenoscope%20Investigation%20FINAL%20Report.pdf. Accessed January 18, 2018.

intended to kill nearly all microbial organisms (except bacterial spores). Critical devices must undergo sterilization, intended to eliminate all microbial life. All endoscopes are considered semicritical devices and should be reprocessed using HLD.[3] The 5 stages of endoscope reprocessing are cleaning, HLD, rinsing, drying, and storage.

For several reasons, semicritical medical devices are far more likely to be associated with disease transmission compared with critical or noncritical devices.[30] Semicritical devices such as endoscopes are often contaminated with a high degree of bacterial bioburden, possess long channels or intricate designs that are challenging to clean, and are prone to biofilm production when moisture is present. Also, as described by Rutala and Weber,[30] any breach in the reprocessing protocol can lead to significant contamination. Specifically, the cleaning step may reduce the bacterial burden by 2 to 6 $\log_{10}$, and HLD may reduce it by an additional 4 to 6 $\log_{10}$, for a total of 6 to 12 $\log_{10}$. Because GI endoscopes may contain 10^{7-10} enteric microorganisms after use, the margin of safety in HLD of GI endoscopes is low to nonexistent, in stark contrast with the 17 $\log_{10}$ margin of safety in sterilization of surgical equipment.[19]

Prompt bioburden removal before HLD is the most important step of reprocessing, because the presence of bioburden impedes the effectiveness of the high-level disinfectant. The cleaning procedure includes precleaning, a leak test, and manual cleaning and reduces the number of microorganisms and organic debris by 4 logs or 99.99%.[10] Manual cleaning of GI endoscopes includes brushing of the external surface and removable parts (eg, suction valves), immersion in an enzymatic detergent solution, followed by irrigation of internal channels with a detergent. Precleaning performed at the point of care immediately after use is emphasized in current guidelines to minimize bioburden drying, which is much more difficult to remove.[3]

The complexity of cleaning places a significant burden on technicians and their supervisors to ensure that every step is done correctly before HLD. Some AERs currently on the market perform automated cleaning in addition to HLD, although they do not replace the initial immediate cleaning step performed at bedside. Although automation provides greater standardization and reduces the risk of human error, the reliability of these devices is yet to be confirmed through independent peer-reviewed studies in clinical settings.

The cleaning process for duodenoscopes, as outlined in the manufacturer instructions for use, is additionally complicated by the need to thoroughly clean the elevator mechanism located at the distal tip of the duodenoscope. These steps may differ depending on the model and type of scope and may change over time as the processes are refined by the FDA and manufacturers.

After cleaning, HLD is performed either through a manual process or via an AER; an AER is preferred when available to standardize the process and the minimize risk of contamination or health care worker exposure to disinfectants.[27]

Disinfectants used for HLD require activity against a broad range of microorganisms and must be used at specific concentration, temperature, and duration for maximal efficacy. Common disinfectants include glutaraldehyde, ortho-phthalaldehyde, and paracetic acid.[6] Glutaraldehyde is commonly used owing to its low cost and noncorrosive activity; however, it is an irritant, requires a long contact time, and resistance has been described in Mycobacteria, Pseudomonas, and other organisms.[10]

After HLD, sterile or filtered water should be used to rinse the endoscope and flush the channels. Ethyl or isopropyl alcohol (70%–90%) should be used to flush the channels, followed by filtered forced air drying.[3] Inadequate drying can facilitate bacterial growth and biofilm formation, and has been associated with outbreaks.[31] Endoscopes should be stored in a manner that protects them from contamination, moisture, or damage. The maximal interval time between use ("shelf life") has not been established, with recommendations ranging from several hours to 21 days or longer.[32] When properly stored, prolonged intervals have not been associated with transmission risk and recent studies demonstrate negligible bacterial contamination after 56 days or longer.[33,34]

Endoscope reprocessing requires meticulous attention to detail and rigid compliance with reprocessing instructions. Unfortunately, lapses are common and frequently implicated in exposure events or outbreaks.[2,6,35] In 2009, the CDC piloted an infection control audit tool during inspection of 68 ambulatory surgical centers in 4 states; compliance with recommendations for reprocessing of endoscopic equipment was found not to be uniform in 28% of 67 ambulatory surgery centers.[36] Given the inherent challenges of endoscope reprocessing and small margin for error, health care workers involved in endoscope reprocessing should receive device-specific training, complete regular competency testing, and undergo routine quality control audits to ensure compliance with all reprocessing guidelines, manufacturer instructions, and institutional policies.[3,30]

RECENT DEVELOPMENTS IN THE PREVENTION OF GASTROINTESTINAL ENDOSCOPE-RELATED INFECTIONS

Based on current understanding, there is an absence of a simple and proven strategy or technology to guarantee patient safety in GI endoscopy infection prevention. Key factors contributing to infection risk from endoscope reprocessing as described by Rutala and Weber are shown in **Table 2**.[37] Recently updated multisociety guidelines provide current recommendations for critical steps in reprocessing flexible GI endoscopes and incorporates guidance specific to duodenoscopes.[3] High compliance with HLD processes is a critical requirement for all endoscopes. For duodenoscopes, all personnel must additionally be trained and knowledgeable in new recommendations for additional flushing and cleaning steps for the elevator channel.[38] User facilities should implement recent interim guidance from the FDA for duodenoscope reprocessing and ensure compliance with updated recommendations as they become available.[39]

Table 2
Factors contributing to infection risk from endoscope reprocessing

Topic	Risk Factor
GI endoscopes are semicritical devices requiring at HLD	Flexible endoscopes are heat labile, so only HLD with chemical agents or low temp sterilization possible (no low temperature sterilizers current FDA cleared for GI endoscopes)
GI endoscopes associated with more outbreaks than any other medical device	Until recent outbreaks, most common sources were deficient practices in cleaning or HLD, damaged endoscopes or design flaws of endoscopes or AERs
Multisociety guidelines developed to assure pathogen-free endoscope	Reliable adherence to all steps of manual endoscope processing per guidelines is challenging
Transmission of infections unrecognized	Inadequate surveillance, long delay from colonization to infection and low frequency of clinical infection
Margin of safety minimal with endoscope reprocessing (vs cleaning/sterilization of surgical instruments)	High microbial burden that can enter internal channels of GI endoscope not amenable to ensuring elimination of organisms after cleaning/HLD

Abbreviations: AER, automated endoscope reprocessor; FDA, US Food and Drug Administration; GI, gastrointestinal; HLD, high-level disinfection.

Data from Rutala WA, Weber DW. Gastrointestinal endoscopes: a need to shift from disinfection to sterilization? JAMA 2014;312(14):1405–6.

In response to the multiple duodenoscope outbreaks, the FDA and CDC outlined 4 optional additional enhanced disinfection measures for consideration by health care providers to decrease the risk of infection and include microbiologic testing of duodenoscopes after processing, ethylene oxide (ETO) sterilization, use of liquid chemical sterilants for HLD, and repeat HLD.[39] It is unclear how many health care facilities have adopted these new processes; however, herein is a description of these enhanced processes, as well as their advantages and disadvantages.

Sterilization

ERCP endoscopes and reusable accessories, such as biopsy forceps, are used in sterile body cavities and as such, many experts consider that they should be classified as critical devices.[37] As stated, the material composition of most flexible endoscopes precludes steam sterilization.

Ethylene oxide

Gas sterilization with ETO has been used for decades to sterilize medical equipment and supplies and is included in reprocessing instructions of many endoscopes. As with all methods of disinfection, ETO is less effective if manual cleaning is not performed well or in the presence of biofilm. Despite the appeal of gas sterilization, many health care facilities have eliminated the use of ETO because of its potential safety risks to employees, given its flammability and carcinogenic potential. At present, prolonged exposure to ETO is the only low-temperature sterilization technique available; however, it is costly, inefficient, associated with potential toxicity to personnel, cannot sterilize residual gross soil, warrants concern about endoscope durability, and is not widely available. Furthermore, ETO is not approved by the FDA for reprocessing endoscopes.[5]

Liquid chemical sterilants

Endoscope processing systems that use liquid chemical sterilants such as peracetic acid are attractive because they are widely accessible within health care facilities, have a decreased turnaround time, and provide a greater safety profile for health care workers. All current duodenoscope manufacturers provide instructions for use with liquid chemical sterilants for either HLD or sterilization. Unfortunately, only 1 liquid chemical sterilant system is currently available in the United States that offers sterilization, Steris System 1e (http://www.steris.com/products/system1e). Because of the risk of exposure to patients, AERs using liquid chemical sterilants require a flush step that uses filtered tap water, which renders the scopes nonsterile at the end of the cycle; it is also unclear whether peracetic acid will penetrate crevices in the duodenoscope elevator channel and inactivate pathogens. Additionally, because many health care facilities currently use AERs that can only operate with aldehyde-based chemistries, capital costs would be incurred for the purchase of new equipment.[5]

Measures of Cleaning Efficacy

The use of real-time monitoring methods has been proposed to assess the effectiveness of cleaning and HLD as well as the risk of infection, yet remain investigational and have not been widely applied in clinical practice.[40] Adenosine triphosphate detection of effluent has been the most widely used and studied for assessing cleaning adequacy before exposure to HLD, because it detects organic residuals. However, adenosine triphosphate is not a good indicator of microbial contamination and has not been validated as a method to assess the risk for patient-to-patient transmission.[19] Nonetheless, the results do seem to correlate with clearance of precleaning and manual cleaning steps. Therefore, this method of assessment of bioburden may be of use in training, competency testing, and random surveillance of the cleaning steps before HLD.[3] Because cleaning is so critical, many health care facilities have adopted a validation step using detection of adenosine triphosphate or protein burden as an additional part of their process, with repeat cleaning of scopes falling outside the acceptable ranges.[1] Additionally, scopes that fail more often than others may signal damaged internal surfaces and trigger service for the scope to ensure it can be cleaned adequately.

Cultures

Routine microbiological testing for endoscopes and AERs remains a controversial issue in many guidelines. Microbiological testing methods, per the CDC's interim surveillance protocol, are based on international experience (Australia and Europe) and were intended for use in health care facilities as part of a quality assurance program.[42] These methods require aseptic microbiologic sampling of each endoscope after processing or at some defined interval, and then holding the endoscopes in quarantine for 48 to 72 hours until microbial growth can be detected (culture and hold). Standardized protocols outlining bacterial growth levels and bacterial identification determine whether the endoscope can be safely used. However, this approach was not widely adopted in the United States largely owing to a lack of data on test characteristics and performance. Recent outbreaks where bacteria were not recovered from epidemiologically implicated duodenoscopes have demonstrated that a negative culture result does not eliminate the respective instrument as a potential source. In addition, the American Society of Microbiology has advised against performance of endoscope cultures by hospital clinical diagnostic laboratory tests out of concern that recipients of negative cultures will misinterpret them as evidence of sterility and from concerns about some technical aspects of the CDC protocol.[19] Although some hospitals have chosen to perform endoscope cultures in their clinical laboratory despite these concerns, other health care facilities have outsourced the testing, adding logistical complexity, cost, and increased endoscope turnaround time.[43] In May 2015, the FDA's Gastroenterology and Urology Devices Panel of the Medical Devices Advisory Committee concluded that the CDC's interim guidance for surveillance for bacterial contamination of duodenoscopes after reprocessing "is not sufficient in the current form to be implemented by health care facilities as a best practice."[44] Although some health care facilities have implemented such a process, many have chosen not to do so owing to the significant resources required (technologist and microbiologist time and requirement for additional endoscopes owing to an increased turnaround time).[43,45]

Repeat High-Level Disinfection

The FDA-recommended practice of performing 2 successive HLD cycles on endoscopes before use is based on a theoretic rationale that back-to-back HLD may reduce or eliminate microbial contaminants remaining from the first cycle. Although this practice has been used in some countries, there is little published evidence to support the practice and it can increase turnaround time. The greatest concern regarding this practice is its lack of efficacy, based on the observation that contaminated duodenoscopes have caused outbreaks at health care facilities throughout the United States and Europe despite having undergone sometimes dozens of cycles of HLD without eradicating the bacteria. This finding suggests that there may be internal bacterial contamination of the duodenoscopes on surfaces that are not adequately disinfected by HLD and therefore not addressed through multiple HLD cycles.

Infection Surveillance

Detection of endoscope related infections remains challenging and current guidelines lack specific guidance on enhanced detection approaches. Although the CDC has a validated system for monitoring surgical site infections after surgery, there is currently no corresponding surveillance approach for detecting infections after endoscopy. Although the small infection risks associated with many types of endoscopy likely render surveillance a low yield activity, in the wake of duodenosope outbreaks at multiple centers, surveillance programs may facilitate the early detection of outbreaks; health care facilities can apply approaches similar to those currently used to identify surgical site infections, using microbiology data and *International Classification of Diseases,* 10th edition, complication codes within 30 days after the procedure. Collecting such surveillance data may provide baseline information regarding complications after duodenoscopy and facilitate opportunities to identify trends or signals that may point to a cluster or outbreak. The low frequency, prolonged incubation period, and potential for unrecognized clinical symptoms in outpatients may pose challenges to a surveillance program for an infrequent occurrence.

Future areas of development for prevention of infections include the redesign of endoscopes by manufacturers (eg, elevator channel) to facilitate optimal HLD or sterilization and the development of single use, sterile disposable GI endoscopes.

SUMMARY

Endoscopy will remain an important diagnostic and therapeutic modality. The recent outbreaks of duodenoscope-related infections have highlighted previously underappreciated risks of infection associated with these procedures and have prompted a broad reevaluation of the methods of cleaning and disinfection of GI endoscopes.

Many issues remain unresolved in the current guidelines owing to the lack of robust data to develop specific recommendations. However, it is clear that compliance with accepted guidelines for the reprocessing of GI endoscopes between patients is critical to the safety and success of their use and that, on the whole, when these guidelines are followed, pathogen transmission can be minimized. Increased efforts and resources should be directed to improve compliance with these guidelines and to future research in prevention of GI endoscope related infections. In the meantime, health care facilities should improve their own internal quality control processes, regularly reinforce necessary competencies, and consider performing postprocedure infection surveillance. Until methods to sterilize these devices can be implemented to ensure optimal patient safety from infection risks associated with GI endoscopy, continued vigilance is required to ensure strict adherence to current reprocessing guidelines and to detect infrequent infections that may signal breaks in adherence to current processes, design flaws that increase risk, or damaged equipment.

REFERENCES

1. Peery AF, Dellon ES, Lund J, et al. Burden of gastrointestinal disease in the United States: 2012 update. Gastroenterology 2012;143(5):1179–87.
2. Humphries RM, McDonnell G. Superbugs on duodenoscopes: the challenges of cleaning and disinfection of resuable devices. J Clin Microbiol 2015;53(10): 3118–25.
3. Petersen BT, Cohen J, Hambrick RD, et al. Multisociety guideline on reprocessing flexible gastrointestinal endoscopes: 2016 update. Gastrointest Endosc 2017; 85(2):282–94.
4. ASGE Standards of Practice Committee, Chandrasekhara V, Khashab MA, Muthusamy VR, et al. Adverse events associated with ERCP. Gastrointest Endosc 2017;85(1):32–47.
5. Rubin ZA, Murthy RK. Outbreaks associated with duodenoscopes: new challenges and controversies. Curr Opin Infect Dis 2016;29.407–14.
6. Kovaleva J, Peters FTM, van der Mei HC, et al. Transmission of infection by flexible gastrointestinal endoscopy and bronchoscopy. Clin Microbiol Rev 2013; 26(2):231–54.
7. US Food and Drug Administration (FDA). Effective reprocessing of endoscopes used in endoscopic retrograde cholangiopancreatography (ERCP) procedures, executive summary 2015. Available at: http://regulatorydoctor.us/wp-content/uploads/2015/07/Effective-Reprocessing-of-Endoscopes-Used-in-ERCP.pdf. Accessed February 17, 2018.
8. Ahmed M, Kanotra R, Savani GT, et al. Utilization trends in inpatient endoscopic retrograde cholangiopancreatography (ERCP): a cross-sectional US experience. Endosc Int Open 2017;5(4):E261–71.
9. Botoman VA, Surawicz CM. Bacteremia with gastrointestinal endoscopic procedures. Gastrointest Endosc 1986;32(5):342–6.
10. Kovaleva J. Infectious Complications in gastrointestinal endoscopy and their prevention. Best Pract Res Clin Gastroenterol 2016;30:689–704.
11. Sung YK, Lee JK, Lee KH, et al. The clinical epidemiology and outcomes of bacteremic biliary tract infections caused by antimicrobial-resistant pathogens. Am J Gastroenterol 2012;107(3):473–83.
12. Babinchak T, Badal R, Hoban D, et al. Trends in susceptibility of selected gram-negative bacilli isolated from intra-abdominal infections in North America: SMART 2005-2010. Diagn Microbiol Infect Dis 2013;76(3):379–81.

13. Jacob JT, Klein E, Laxminarayan, et al. Vital signs: carbapenem-resistant entero-bacteriaceae. MMWR Morb Mortal Wkly Rep 2013;62(9):165–70.
14. Rutala WA, Weber DJ. Healthcare infection control practices advisory committee. Guideline for disinfection and sterilization in healthcare facilities, 2008. Available at: http://www.cdc.gov/ncidod/dhqp/pdf/guidelines/Disinfection_Nov_2008.pdf. Accessed February 10 2018.
15. Muscarella LF. Risk of transmission of carbapenem-resistant Enterobacteriaceae and related "superbugs" during gastrointestinal endoscopy. World J Gastrointest Endosc 2014;6(10):457–74.
16. Centers for Disease Control and Prevention (CDC). Infectious disease antibiotic resistance threats in the United States, 2013. Available at: https://www.cdc.gov/drugresistance/pdf/ar-threats-2013-508.pdf. Accessed February 16, 2018.
17. Epstein L, Hunter JC, Arwady MA, et al. New Delhi metallo-b-lactamase–producing carbapenem-resistant Escherichia coli associated with exposure to duodeno-scopes. JAMA 2014;312:1447–55.
18. Yang D, Zhang Z. Biofilm-forming Klebsiella pneumoniae strains have greater likelihood of producing extended-spectrum b-lactamases. J Hosp Infect 2008; 68:369–71.
19. Rutala WA, Weber DJ. ERCP scopes: what can we do to prevent infections? Infect Control Hosp Epidemiol 2015;36:643–8.
20. Kimmey MB, Burnett DA, Carr-Locke DL, et al. Transmission of infection by gastrointestinal endoscopy. Gastrointest Endosc 1993;39:885–8.
21. Seoane-Vazquez E, Rodriguez-Monguio R, Visaria J, et al. Exogenous endoscopy-related infections, pseudo-infections, and toxic reactions: clinical and economic burden. Curr Med Res Opin 2006;22(10):2007–21.
22. Nelson DB, Muscarella LF. Current issues in endoscope reprocessing and infection control during gastrointestinal endoscopy. World J Gastroenterol 2006; 12(25):3953–64.
23. Alvarado CJ, Stolz SM, Maki DG. Nosocomial infections from contaminated endo-scopes: a flawed automated endoscope washer. An investigation using molecular epidemiology. Am J Med 1991;91(3B):272S–80S.
24. Allen JI, Allen MO, Olson MM, et al. Pseudomonas infection of the biliary system resulting from use of a contaminated endoscope. Gastroenterology 1987;92: 759–63.
25. ASGE Technology Committee, Parsi MA, Sullivan SA, Goodman A, et al. Auto-mated endoscope reprocessors. Gastrointest Endosc 2016;84(6):885–92.
26. Hervé RC, Keevil CW. Persistent residual contamination in endoscope channels; a fluorescence epimicroscopy study. Endoscopy 2016;48(7):609–16.
27. Petersen BT, Chennat J, Cohen J, et al. Multisociety guideline on reprocessing flexible GI endoscopes: 2011. Infect Control Hosp Epidemiol 2011;32(6): 527–37.
28. US Senate. Senate Health, education, labor and pensions committee & minority staff report: preventable tragedies: superbugs and how ineffective monitoring of medical device safety fails patients. Patty Murray, ranking member Jan 13, 2016. Available at: https://www.help.senate.gov/imo/media/doc/Duodenoscope %20Investigation%20FINAL%20Report.pdf. Accessed January 18, 2018.
29. Rutala WA, Weber DJ. Disinfection and sterilization in health care facilities: what clinicians need to know. Clin Infect Dis 2004;39:702–9.
30. Rutala WA, Weber DJ. Reprocessing semicritical items: current issues and new technologies. Am J Infect Control 2016;44:e53–62.

31. Muscarella LF. Inconsistencies in endoscope-reprocessing and infection-control guidelines: the importance of endoscope drying. Am J Gastroenterol 2006; 101(9):2147–54.

32. Bashaw MA. Guideline Implementation: processing flexible endoscopes. AORN J 2016;104:226–33.

33. Scanlon P, Flaherty K, Reilly EA, et al. Association between storage interval and contamination of reprocessed flexible endoscopes in a pediatric gastrointestinal procedural unit. Infect Control Hosp Epidemiol 2017;38(2):131–5.

34. Mallette KI, Pieroni P, Dhalla SS. Bacterial presence on flexible endoscopes vs time since disinfection. World J Gastrointest Endosc 2018;10(1):51–5.

35. Dirlam Langlay AM, Ofstead CL, Mueller NJ, et al. Reported gastrointestinal endoscope reprocessing lapses: the tip of the iceberg. Am J Infect Control 2013;41:1188–94.

36. Schaefer MK, Jhung M, Dahl M, et al. Infection control assessment of ambulatory surgical centers. JAMA 2010;303:2273–9.

37. Rutala WA, Weber DW. Gastrointestinal endoscopes: a need to shift from disinfection to sterilization? JAMA 2014;312(14):1405–6.

38. New reprocessing instructions for the Olympus TJF Q180V duodenoscope. Olympus America website. 2015. Available at: http://medical. olympusamerica. com/sites/default/files/pdf/150326_TJF-Q180V_Customer_letter.pdf). Available at: http://medical.olympusamerica.com/sites/default/files/pdf/150326_TJF-Q180V_ Customer_letter.pdf. Accessed March 27, 2015.

39. Food and Drug Administration (FDA). Supplemental measures to enhance duodeno-scope reprocessing: FDA safety communication. 2015. Available at: https:// wayback.archive-it.org/7993/20170722150658/https://www.fda.gov/MedicalDevices/ Safety/AlertsandNotices/ucm454766.htm. Accessed February 19, 2018.

40. Petersen BT. Monitoring of endoscope reprocessing: accumulating data but best practices remain undefined. Infect Control Hosp Epidemiol 2014;35: 995–7.

41. Fushimi R, Takashina M, Yoshikawa H, et al. Comparison of adenosine triphos-phate, microbiological load, and residual protein as indicators for assessing the cleanliness of flexible gastrointestinal endoscopes. Am J Infect Control 2013;41(2):161–4.

42. Centers for Disease Control and Prevention (CDC). Interim protocol for healthcare facilities regarding surveillance for bacterial contamination of duodenoscopes after reprocessing. Available at: https://www.cdc.gov/hai/pdfs/cre/interim-duodenoscope-surveillance-Protocol.pdf. Accessed January 25, 2018.

43. Ross AS, Baliga C, Verma P, et al. A quarantine process for the resolution of duodenoscope-associated transmission of multidrug resistant Escherichia coli. Gastrointest Endosc 2015;82:477–83.

44. Food and Drug Administration (FDA). Brief summary of the gastroenterology and urology devices panel meeting, May 14–15, 2015. Available at: http://www.fda. gov/downloads/AdvisoryCommittees/CommitteesMeetingMaterials/MedicalDevices/ MedicalDevicesAdvisory Committee/Gastroenterology-UrologyDevicesPanel/ UCM447407.pdf. Accessed February 12, 2018.

45. Almario C, May FP, Shaheen NJ, et al. Cost utility of competing strategies to pre-vent endoscopic transmission of carbapenem-resistant enterobacteriaceae. Am J Gastroenterol 2015;110:1666–74.

46. Verfaillie C, Bruno MJ, Voor in't Holt AF, et al. Withdrawal of a novel-design duo-denoscope ends outbreak of a VIM-2-producing Pseudomonas aeruginosa. Endoscopy 2015;47:493–502.

47. McCool S, Clarke L, Querry A, et al. Carbapenem-resistant Enterobacteriaceae (CRE) Klebsiella pneumonia (KP) cluster analysis associated with GI scopes with elevator channel. Presented at ID Week. San Francisco, California, October 2–6, 2013. [abstract: 1619].

48. Kola A, Piening B, Pape UF, et al. An outbreak of carbapenem-resistant OXA-48-producing Klebsiella pneumonia associated to duodenoscopy. Antimicrob Resist Infect Control 2015;4:8.

49. Smith ZL, Young SO, Saeian K, et al. Transmission of carbapenem-resistant Enterobacteriaciae during ERCP: time to revisit the current reprocessing guidelines. Gastrointest Endosc 2015;81:1041–5.

50. Wendorf K, Kay M, Baliga C, et al. Endoscopic retrograde cholangiopancreatography-associated AmpC Escherichia coli outbreak. Infect Control Hosp Epidemiol 2015; 36(6):634–42.

51. Available at: https://www.cedars-sinai.edu/About-Us/News/News-Releases-2015/Media-Statement-Regarding-CRE-and-Duodenoscope.aspx. Accessed February 17, 2018.

52. Available at: https://www.uclahealth.org/ucla-statement-on-notification-of-patients-regarding-endoscopic-procedures. Accessed February 17, 2018.

Understanding Biofilms and Novel Approaches to the Diagnosis, Prevention, and Treatment of Medical Device-Associated Infections

Yu Mi Wi, MD, PhD[a], Robin Patel, MD[b,c,*]

KEYWORDS

- Biofilm • Extracellular polymeric substance • Tolerance
- Medical device-associated infection • Surface-coating or eluting substrate
- Physical–mechanical approach • Extracellular polymeric substance targeting therapy

KEY POINTS

- Treatment of device-related infections is challenging because microorganisms adhere to and accumulate on the surfaces of medical devices producing biofilms.
- The viable but nonculturable state and emergence of small colony variants can render successful diagnosis of biofilm-associated infections difficult using standard microbiological assays.
- Sonication of infected implants and molecular diagnostic methods may not only improve detection and identification of pathogens but also reveal greater microbial diversity than standard microbiological assays.
- Surface-coating or eluting substrates and physical/mechanical/electrical/biological approaches are in use and/or under development for inhibition of initial bacterial attachment and for bacterial removal.
- Recent advances in surface technologies and materials have ushered in material optimization and surface modification with antifouling polyurethanes, hydrogels, and bacteriophages.
- Recent insights into biofilm matrix have accelerated novel biofilm-targeting therapeutic strategies.

Financial Disclosures: See last page of article.
[a] Division of Infectious Diseases, Department of Internal Medicine, Samsung Changwon Hospital, Sungkyunkwan University, 158 palyong-ro, MasanHoiwon-gu, Changwon-si, Gyeongsangnam-do 51353, Korea; [b] Division of Clinical Microbiology, Department of Laboratory Medicine and Pathology, Mayo Clinic, 200 First Street Southwest, Rochester, MN 55905, USA; [c] Division of Infectious Diseases, Department of Medicine, Mayo Clinic, 200 First Street Southwest, Rochester, MN 55905, USA
* Corresponding author. Division of Clinical Microbiology, Department of Laboratory Medicine and Pathology, Mayo Clinic, 200 First Street Southwest, Rochester, MN 55905.
E-mail address: robin.patel@mayo.edu

Infect Dis Clin N Am 32 (2018) 915–929
https://doi.org/10.1016/j.idc.2018.06.009
id.theclinics.com

INTRODUCTION

Medical device-associated infections are one of the most common and feared complications in medical practice. The treatment of medical device-related infections is notoriously challenging and recurrence is common.[1] The main reason for this situation is that microorganisms adhere to the surfaces of medical devices and enter into a biofilm state in which they display distinct structural features, growth rates, and microenvironments, when compared with planktonic organisms.[2,3] A decreased susceptibility to antimicrobial agents and the host immune system is observed in microorganisms in biofilms compared with planktonically grown organisms.[4] The biofilm structure itself, decreased growth rate, antimicrobial-destroying enzymes within the matrix, upregulation of stress response genes, and horizontal transfer of antimicrobial resistance genes are involved in decreased antimicrobial susceptibility.[3,4] Microorganisms in mature biofilms more than 7 day old are 500 to 5000 times less susceptible to killing by many antimicrobial agents compared with planktonic organisms.[5]

Many controversies and uncertainties exist in the diagnosis, prevention, and treatment of biofilm-associated infection.[6] Once a biofilm develops on a medical device, the eradication of microorganisms becomes extremely challenging and cost can be substantial owing to the frequent need for prolonged hospitalization, surgery, and long-term antimicrobial treatment.[7] Bacterial biofilms are associated with approximately 1.7 million hospital-acquired infections annually in the United States, incurring an annual economic burden of approximately $11 billion.[8] Biofilm formation is now accepted as one of the most important virulence factors in medical device-associated infections.[2]

This article reviews the means by which microorganisms form biofilms, and how biofilms provide protection against the host immune system and antimicrobial agents. Also discussed are innovative concepts for the diagnosis of biofilm-associated infection and novel approaches to treatment and prevention of medical device-associated infections.

UNDERSTANDING OF BIOFILMS
Definition and Structure of Biofilms

Biofilms appear very early in the fossil record and can be formed by a diverse range of microorganisms; they are widespread in natural, industrial, and hospital settings.[9] A biofilm is generally defined as an aggregate of microorganisms adherent to a biotic or abiotic surface, embedded within a matrix of extracellular polymeric substance (EPS; **Fig. 1**).[10] Interestingly, free-floating cells can also self-aggregate and form a biofilm, which can display features similar to those of a medical device-associated biofilm.[10,11] A major feature of biofilms is their self-produced EPS, which consists of polysaccharides, nucleic acids, and/or proteins.[3] The EPS matrix advances microbial attachment to surfaces and cell-to-cell adhesion and aggregation and functions as a 3-dimensional barrier to protect cells against from external threats, including host defense mechanisms and antimicrobial treatment.[12] Moreover, the EPS matrix can create harsh environments by modulating chemical and nutrient gradients, and contribute to important virulence attributes.[12] Host-derived components, including fibrin, platelets, and immunoglobulins, may also be components of biofilms in complex host environments. A description of biofilms as aggregated, microbial cells surrounded by a polymeric self-produced matrix, which may contain host components was suggested at the 5th American Society for Microbiology Biofilm Conference.[10] Microorganisms can attach to almost all types of medical devices and also biotic surfaces (eg, skin, bone, airway mucosa, connective tissue, intestinal mucosa, and vascular endothelium).[9] Therefore, biofilms may be associated with various types of

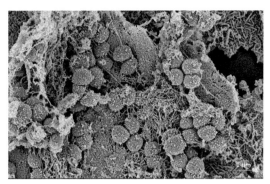

Fig. 1. Scanning electron microscopy of *Staphylococcus epidermidis* biofilm. *S epidermidis* was grown in the laboratory on a Teflon surface.

tissue-associated chronic infections, in addition to their association with medical devices (**Table 1**). Medical device-associated infections are most commonly caused by *Staphylococcus epidermidis* and *Staphylococcus aureus*, but a long list of species of bacteria and fungi can cause these infections.[13,14] Although some authors suggest that staphylococci account the majority of the bacteria causing medical device-related infections,[15] in the hospital setting, multidrug-resistant gram-negative bacteria such as *Escherichia coli*, *Klebsiella pneumoniae, Acinetobacter baumannii*, and *Pseudomonas aeruginosa* have emerged as serious concerns, especially in catheter-associated urinary tract infections.[16]

Stages of Biofilms

The initial step of biofilm formation is initiated by complex interactions between surfaces and the microorganism (or microorganisms). Biofilm formation consists of several stages, beginning with attachment and progressing to detachment (**Fig. 2**).[2] At the stage of initial attachment, surface characteristics such as hydrophobicity, charge, topography, and exposure time influence the attachment of microorganisms to the surface of medical devices.[17] Adherence of microorganisms to medical devices has been reported to occur through cell surface proteins, such as biofilm-associated protein—a fimbria-like polymer—, the protein autolysin of *S*

Table 1	
Biofilm-associated infections	
Medical Devices Associated with Infections	**Tissues Associated with Infections**
Cardiovascular implantable electronic devices	Biliary tract
Catheters, shunts, and stents	Internal ear (chronic otitis media)
Cochlear implants	Tonsils (chronic tonsillitis)
Contact lenses	Sinuses (chronic sinusitis)
Deep brain stimulators	Wounds
Endotracheal tubes	Teeth (dental caries)
Dental implants	Heart valves (endocarditis)
Orthopedic implants	Kidney stones
Tissue fillers, including breast implants	Lung (cystic fibrosis patients)
Sutures and surgical meshes	Bone (osteomyelitis)
Vascular grafts	

Data from Hoiby N, Bjarnsholt T, Moser C, et al. ESCMID guideline for the diagnosis and treatment of biofilm infections 2014. Clin Microbiol Infect 2015;21 Suppl 1:S1–25.

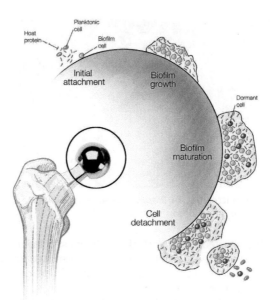

Fig. 2. Steps in biofilm formation on an orthopedic prosthesis. Biofilm formation has distinct stages: initial attachment, in which microorganism attaches to an orthopedic implant through interactions between the microorganism and host molecules on the foreign body surface as well as the foreign body surface itself; biofilm growth, in which the microorganism begins to proliferate, and individual cells adhere to one another and become surrounded by a self-produced extracellular polymeric substance; biofilm maturation, whereby the biofilm develops a structured multicellular community protecting its members from external threats, including host defense mechanisms and antimicrobial treatments; and finally cell detachment, whereby planktonic cells may be released from the surface of large biofilms, causing distant metastatic infections and further regional biofilm establishment.

epidermidis, and the capsular polysaccharide/adhesion of *S epidermidis* and other coagulase-negative staphylococci.[18–21] Host-derived proteins, such as fibronectin, fibrinogen, and vitronectin, released to aid in healing, are absorbed onto the surfaces of medical devices, producing a conditioning film that enhances microbial colonization through interactions between microbial and host proteins.[17,18] At the stage of biofilm growth, microorganisms proliferate and cell-to-cell adhesion on the colonized surface is enhanced. These organized structures are then surrounded by a self-produced EPS.[2,3,8] As biofilms mature, they become a structured multicellular community providing protection against from external threats, including host defense mechanisms and antimicrobial treatment. Microorganisms in biofilms release autoregulators and have altered gene expression that stimulates the production of virulence factors, enhancing their own survival.[22] At the stage of cell detachment, planktonic cells may be released from the surface, potentially resulting in distant metastatic infections and/or further regional biofilm formation. Dispersed microorganisms revert to an active state, comparable with that of their planktonic counterparts, making them more susceptible to antimicrobial agents.[23] In addition, dispersed biofilm cells lose the protective effects granted by the biofilm community and its structured organization. The cyclic di-GMP second messenger reported in *E coli*, *P aeruginosa*, and *Salmonella enterica*[24] is an example of a molecule responsible for biofilm dispersal.[25]

Tolerance and Resistance of Microorganisms in Biofilms

Biofilm-associated infections are particularly challenging to treat. Several mechanisms account for protection against the host immune system and antimicrobial agents, compared with microorganisms in the planktonic state. This type of resistance is not mainly due to the genetic antimicrobial resistance that occurs by mutation or horizontal gene transfer, but is rather better described as a reversible tolerance to antimicrobial agents.[4,26] Tolerance can be the result of entrapment or inactivation of antimicrobials, and/or of the slow growth that is characteristic of biofilms.[4,26] Restricted penetration of antimicrobial agents into the depth of a mature biofilm owing to the EPS matrix of the biofilm itself can contribute to the antimicrobial tolerance.[4,26] The EPS matrix has also been shown to inactivate antimicrobial substances by harboring enzymes secreted into it.[4,26] Another mechanism involves slow-growing or nongrowing microorganisms owing to nutrient and oxygen depletion within biofilms, particularly with regard to resistance to killing by growth-dependent antimicrobial agents.[9] This phenomenon can be amplified by the presence of phenotypic variants or persister cells.[27] Persister cells are thought to be tolerant to antimicrobial agents because they are in a particularly dormant state.[28] Importantly, dispersed planktonic microorganisms can lose tolerance and restore their susceptibility to antimicrobial agents; thus, targeting dispersal mechanisms is a potential adjuvant strategy to render conventional antimicrobial agents active against biofilms.[29] Growth within a biofilm may facilitate the acquisition of genetic changes such as mutations and gene transfer.[30,31] One study showed that plasmid conjugation was up to 700-fold more efficient in biofilms compared with free-living microorganisms.[32] Similarly, hypermutability may occur in biofilms, with mutation rates for *S aureus* and *S epidermidis* being 4- and 60-fold higher, respectively, in biofilms than that under planktonic conditions.[31] Together, increased gene transfer and hypermutability can increase selection of genetic antimicrobial resistance.

DIAGNOSIS OF MEDICAL DEVICE-ASSOCIATED INFECTIONS

Bearing in mind that most medical device-associated infections are associated with biofilms on the surfaces of the devices, diagnostic strategies that approach the surface of the device are preferred. Sampling surfaces of medical devices may require invasive procedures such as aspiration, biopsy, or extirpation of medical devices. However, device removal is not necessarily required for diagnosis in all situations. For central-line associated bloodstream infections (CLABSI), diagnostic methods based on qualitative (or quantitative) blood cultures, including differential time to positivity, may be used.[33–35] Swab cultures are not recommended because of the small volume of sample available for culture; negative results do not necessarily correlate with the absence of infection.[36] Nevertheless, for some medical device-associate infections, microorganisms may not be identified until the medical device is removed. Moreover, culture is not always positive even when the device is removed. Slow growth rates in biofilms can lead to the viable but nonculturable state microorganisms.[37] *S aureus*, for example, can enter the viable but nonculturable state in biofilms, rendering it undetectable using standard growth media[38]; daptomycin and vancomycin are particularly noteworthy for inducing a viable but nonculturable state in *S aureus* biofilms.[39] The emergence of small colony variants can also render successful diagnosis difficult.[40,41] Small colony variants are slow-growing subpopulations of microorganisms that differ from normal microorganisms in their small colonial size and biochemical characteristics.[41,42] *S aureus* small colony variants have increased intracellular persistence[41] (**Box 1**).

> **Box 1**
> **Clinical features of medical device-associated infections**
>
> - Presence of an indwelling medical device
> - Clinical findings suggestive of infection, often with low-grade inflammation
> - Infection lasting more than 1 week
> - Failure of antibiotic treatment without planktonic genetic antimicrobial resistance
> - Recurrence of infection (particularly if same microorganism is detected over multiple time points, and clinical findings improve/resolve with antibiotic therapy, only to recur after therapy has ceased)
>
> *Data from* Hoiby N, Bjarnsholt T, Moser C, et al. ESCMID guideline for the diagnosis and treatment of biofilm infections 2014. Clin Microbiol Infect 2015;21 Suppl 1:S1–25.

Sonication may improve culture positivity of large device-related infections.[43] One study, focusing on prosthetic hip and knee infections, demonstrated that sonicate fluid cultures had a sensitivity of 79% compared with 61% for periprosthetic tissue cultures.[43] Sonication is not, however, recommended for all devices; the use of a quantitative sonication technique to detect catheter colonization has been shown to be no better than the easier to perform semiquantitative roll-plate culture method.[44] Combinations of sonication with certain nucleic acid amplification tests may further enhance the sensitivity to diagnose infection.[45,46] Several studies show differences between findings using culture and molecular diagnostic methods; molecular methods may identify additional organisms (ie, increased diversity) compared with culture and/or may detect microorganisms in culture-negative cases.[47,48] In culture-negative endocarditis, for example, identification of the causative bacterium by broad-range bacterial (eg, 16S ribosomal RNA gene) polymerase chain reaction of heart valve tissues can be useful.[49] Some infections may be missed or their microbiology not defined because of a high rate of false-negative microbiological results with conventional culture methods; an example is arthroplasty failure.[50–52] As mentioned elsewhere in this article, implant sonication can improve diagnosis. Alternatively, DL-dithiothreitol has been used for detection of biofilms on orthopedic implants.[53] Disclosing agents have been suggested as an intraoperative strategy to visualize biofilms, but the sensitivity of this approach is not defined.[54] Confocal laser scanning microscopy and scanning electron microscopy are advanced options to visualize biofilms in resected specimens,[55,56] but are not typically used in direct patient care.

TREATMENT AND PREVENTION OF MEDICAL DEVICE-ASSOCIATED INFECTIONS

The basic principles of infection prevention should be applied to prevent microbial contamination of implanted devices because, as mentioned, this can readily lead to biofilm formation. Device implantation and handling must be performed as outlined in current guidelines.[57] Appropriate perioperative antibiotic prophylaxis should be administered to cases of surgically implanted devices. And, of course, the need for the indwelling medical device itself must be justifiable at any time.

Current preventive (and to some extent therapeutic) approaches can be divided into 2 broad categories, namely, surface coating or eluting substrates and physical/mechanical/electrical/biological approaches. Surface modification of medical devices using antibiotics and silver has been the focus of much research to decrease microbial colonization and biofilm formation.[1,2,6,58] Minocycline-rifampin catheters, which are commercially available, have been associated with decreases in microbial colonization and CLABSI.[59] Impregnated and standard catheters have similar CLABSI risks over first 10 days after placement, a cost-effectiveness analysis suggested minocycline-rifampin catheters to be most attractive if the catheter is anticipated to be in place for 8 days or more.[60] Chlorhexidine-silver sulfadiazine catheters also decrease microbial colonization of surfaces.[61] Antibiotic impregnated materials may reduce the incidence of orthopedic foreign body-associated infections.[62] A silver-impregnated endotracheal tube showed a maximal effect during the first 10 days of intubation and reduced mortality in patients with ventilator-associated pneumonia.[63] Water sprays and jets have been used as physical–mechanical approaches for biofilm removal (eg, debridement of surgical sites, exudates, or dental biofilms).[64] In addition, the use of dedicated devices to mechanically remove endotracheal tube biofilm is supported by a limited number of studies.[65] Electrical and electrochemical strategies are being investigated as strategies to prevent biofilm formation on device surfaces.[66]

When confronted with therapeutic difficulties, the removal of the indwelling medical device is a definitive option for curing a medical device-associated infection. However, removal of a medical device may not always be feasible or desirable and the removal procedure itself may be prone to complications and associated with substantial costs. Microorganisms in biofilms show a wide degree of tolerance to different antimicrobial agents. Antibiotics such as rifampin, for the staphylococci in particular, and the fluoroquinolones, may exhibit activity.[67,68] Conversely, antibiotics that inhibit cell wall synthesis (eg, β-lactams) may be less active because microorganisms in biofilms display slow growth rates.[69] When using rifampin-based therapy, combination with another antimicrobial agent, rather than monotherapy, must be used to minimize the emergence of rifampin resistance. Glycopeptides or linezolid when combined with rifampin showed enhanced effects against staphylococcal biofilms.[67,70] In a cage-associated methicillin-resistant *S aureus* infection model in guinea pigs, the combination of levofloxacin or daptomycin with rifampin had higher activity than the combination of vancomycin or linezolid with rifampin.[71] Rifampin and fosfomycin or tedizolid also showed enhanced effects in treating medical device infections caused by methicillin-resistant *S aureus* biofilms in vivo.[72,73] Dalbavancin alone has recently been shown to have in vitro activity against staphylococcal and enterococcal biofilms, potentially providing an option to treat dalbavancin-susceptible staphylococcal and enterococcal biofilm-associated infections.[74,75] Oritavancin also demonstrates activity against staphylococcal biofilms.[76] The age of the biofilm and biofilm species composition are important variables that impact susceptibility microorganisms in biofilms. The age of *S epidermidis* biofilms was shown to be related with activity of erythromycin, clindamycin, cephalothin, teicoplanin, and vancomycin.[77] With respect to biofilm species composition, the susceptibility of *Streptococcus pneumoniae* to β-lactam antibiotics was decreased by the co-presence of β-lactamase–producing *Moraxella catarrhalis* in the biofilm.[78] In a biofilm composed of *Candida albicans* and *S epidermidis* combined, the staphylococcal EPS inhibited azole penetration into the biofilm and *C albicans* seemed to protect *S epidermidis* against vancomycin.[79] High dosages of antibiotics and prolonged duration of treatment are also important when treating medical device-associated infections. The application of catheter lock solutions is a strategy to eradicate established biofilm in the catheter lumen; using this approach, antimicrobial agents dwell at supratherapeutic concentrations (sufficient to exhibit antibiofilm activity) in the catheter lumen for a prolonged time. Antimicrobial lock solutions have been shown to decrease the risk of CLABSI in immunocompromised hematologic patients and those undergoing hemodialysis.[80,81] Antibiotic lock therapy is used in conjunction with systemic antibiotics in the treatment of patients with uncomplicated CLABSI.[82]

Recent advances in surface technologies and materials have ushered in development of surface patterns of defined chemistry and topography that can impact biofilm formation without adding antimicrobial agents.[58] Novel materials such as zinconium oxide and electropolished stainless steel reduce bacterial adhesion.[27] Incorporation of the Sharklet micropattern (patterned after shark skin) on the surface of medical devices may decrease microbial colonization and biofilm formation.[83] Several studies show the feasibility and efficacy of surface modification of medical devices with antifouling polyurethanes and hydrogels to reduce microbial colonization.[1,27] Bacteriophages are viruses that propagate in their bacterial host, and can kill their host and/or produce antibiofilm substances.[84] Pretreating hydrogel-coated catheters with a single S epidermidis bacteriophage or a cocktail of P aeruginosa bacteriophages mitigated biofilm formation by relevant bacteria in vitro.[85–87]

Recent insights into the complexity of biofilm biology have informed the development of novel biofilm-targeting therapeutic strategies.[1,2,27] EPS-degrading enzymes are a new strategy that may enhance efficacy of antimicrobial agents against biofilms.[88,89] Enzymes such as deoxyribonuclease and dispersin B may be useful adjuvants in this regard.[88,89] Both deoxyribonuclease and dispersin B are being investigated as promising options for biomedical coatings.[90] Another antibiofilm strategy is the use of lysins—bacteriophage-encoded peptidoglycan hydrolases.[91] Small molecules such as mannosides or peptides impede bacterial adhesin binding to host surfaces, thereby preventing biofilm formation.[92–94] The widespread use of quorum sensing systems of bacteria for controlling virulence and biofilm formation constitutes another tactic for the development of novel therapeutics.[95] Nanoparticles provide yet[96] another exciting area of development of new biofilm-targeting methodologies. Nanoparticles are currently in the spotlight mainly for their intrinsic antimicrobial activity and antibiofilm potential together with relatively low toxicity to the host.[97] Nanoparticles can be used for the targeted delivery of antibacterial and antibiofilm agents.[98] Liposomes are widely used as representative organic nanoparticles for delivery of antimicrobial agents.[99–103] Recently, nanomodified endotracheal tubes have been shown to have decreased bacterial colonization compared with unmodified endotracheal tubes.[104,105] Nano- and chemical engineering approaches can be used to develop improved materials for prevention of biofilm formation. Finally, electrical and electrochemical strategies are being developed for their antibiofilm activities.[96,106–114]

SUMMARY

Medical device-associated infections are biofilm-associated infections related to organized communities of microorganisms embedded within a matrix of EPS of microbial and host origin. Because of the entrapment or inactivation of antimicrobial agents, and of the slow growth in biofilms, microorganisms in biofilms display tolerance to a wide range of antimicrobial agents. The viable but nonculturable state and emergence of small colony variants in biofilms can make successful diagnosis difficult using standard microbiological assays. New diagnostic techniques such as sonication of large implants and molecular diagnostic methods may improve not only identification of pathogens, but also reveal greater microbial diversity than previously appreciated. Although most currently available antibiotics have poor activity against microorganisms in biofilms, some, notably rifampin against staphylococci, have been shown to be active against biofilms. Surface-coating or eluting substrates and physical/mechanical/chemical/electrical/biological approaches aimed at inhibition of initial attachment and biofilm removal are two current biofilm-targeting approaches under development. Recent advances in surface technologies and materials have ushered in material optimization and surface modification with antifouling polyurethanes, hydrogels, and bacteriophages. Recent insights into the biofilm matrix have accelerated novel biofilm-targeting therapeutic strategies such as EPS-degrading enzymes, small molecules targeting host–EPS interactions, and quorum sensing systems involved in biofilm formation and dispersal. Electrical and electrochemical strategies are under development.

FINANCIAL DISCLOSURES

Dr R. Patel reports grants from CD Diagnostics, BioFire, Curetis, Merck, Hutchison Biofilm Medical Solutions, Accelerate Diagnostics, Allergan, and The Medicines Company. Dr R. Patel is or has been a consultant to Curetis, Qvella, St. Jude, Beckman Coulter, Morgan Stanley, Heraeus Medical GmbH, CORMATRIX, Specific Technologies, Diaxonit, Selux Dx, GenMark Diagnostics, LBT Innovations Ltd, PathoQuest and Genentech; monies are paid to Mayo Clinic. In addition, Dr R. Patel has a patent on *Bordetella pertussis/parapertussis* polymerase chain reaction issued, a patent on a device/method for sonication with royalties paid by Samsung to Mayo Clinic, and a patent on an antibiofilm substance issued. Dr R. Patel has served on an Actelion data monitoring board. Dr R. Patel receives travel reimbursement from the American Society for Microbiology (ASM) and Infectious Diseases Society of America (IDSA) and an editor's stipend from the ASM and IDSA, and honoraria from the National Board of Medical Examiners, Up-to-Date, and the Infectious Diseases Board Review Course. Dr Y.M. Wi has nothing to disclose. This publication was supported by the National Institutes of Health under award numbers R01 AR056647, R01 AI091594, and R21 AI125870. The content is solely the responsibility of the authors and does not necessarily represent the official views of the National Institutes of Health.

REFERENCES

1. Percival SL, Suleman L, Vuotto C, et al. Healthcare-associated infections, medical devices and biofilms: risk, tolerance and control. J Med Microbiol 2015; 64(Pt 4):323–34.
2. Koo H, Allan RN, Howlin RP, et al. Targeting microbial biofilms: current and prospective therapeutic strategies. Nat Rev Microbiol 2017;15(12):740–55.
3. Flemming HC, Wingender J, Szewzyk U, et al. Biofilms: an emergent form of bacterial life. Nat Rev Microbiol 2016;14(9):563–75.
4. Brauner A, Fridman O, Gefen O, et al. Distinguishing between resistance, tolerance and persistence to antibiotic treatment. Nat Rev Microbiol 2016;14(5): 320–30.
5. Khoury AE, Lam K, Ellis B, et al. Prevention and control of bacterial infections associated with medical devices. ASAIO J 1992;38(3):M174–8.
6. Hoiby N, Bjarnsholt T, Moser C, et al. ESCMID guideline for the diagnosis and treatment of biofilm infections 2014. Clin Microbiol Infect 2015;21(Suppl 1): S1–25.
7. Crowe JF, Sculco TP, Kahn B. Revision total hip arthroplasty: hospital cost and reimbursement analysis. Clin Orthop Relat Res 2003;(413):175–82.
8. Romling U, Kjelleberg S, Normark S, et al. Microbial biofilm formation: a need to act. J Intern Med 2014;276(2):98–110.

9. Hall-Stoodley L, Costerton JW, Stoodley P. Bacterial biofilms: from the natural environment to infectious diseases. Nat Rev Microbiol 2004;2(2):95–108.

10. Hall-Stoodley L, Stoodley P, Kathju S, et al. Towards diagnostic guidelines for biofilm-associated infections. FEMS Immunol Med Microbiol 2012;65(2):127–45.

11. Perez K, Patel R. Biofilm-like aggregation of *Staphylococcus epidermidis* in synovial fluid. J Infect Dis 2015;212(2):335–6.

12. Hobley L, Harkins C, MacPhee CE, et al. Giving structure to the biofilm matrix: an overview of individual strategies and emerging common themes. FEMS Microbiol Rev 2015;39(5):649–69.

13. Becker K, Heilmann C, Peters G. Coagulase-negative staphylococci. Clin Microbiol Rev 2014;27(4):870–926.

14. Gotz F. Staphylococcus and biofilms. Mol Microbiol 2002;43(6):1367–78.

15. von Eiff C, Heilmann C, Peters G. New aspects in the molecular basis of polymer-associated infections due to staphylococci. Eur J Clin Microbiol Infect Dis 1999;18(12):843–6.

16. Niveditha S, Pramodhini S, Umadevi S, et al. The isolation and the biofilm formation of uropathogens in the patients with catheter associated urinary tract infections (UTIs). J Clin Diagn Res 2012;6(9):1478–82.

17. Rochford ET, Richards RG, Moriarty TF. Influence of material on the development of device-associated infections. Clin Microbiol Infect 2012;18(12):1162–7.

18. Heilmann C, Hussain M, Peters G, et al. Evidence for autolysin-mediated primary attachment of *Staphylococcus epidermidis* to a polystyrene surface. Mol Microbiol 1997;24(5):1013–24.

19. Hagihara M, Crandon JL, Nicolau DP. The efficacy and safety of antibiotic combination therapy for infections caused by Gram-positive and Gram-negative organisms. Expert Opin Drug Saf 2012;11(2):221–33.

20. Muller E, Hubner J, Gutierrez N, et al. Isolation and characterization of transposon mutants of *Staphylococcus epidermidis* deficient in capsular polysaccharide/adhesin and slime. Infect Immun 1993;61(2):551–8.

21. Veenstra GJ, Cremers FF, van Dijk H, et al. Ultrastructural organization and regulation of a biomaterial adhesin of Staphylococcus epidermidis. J Bacteriol 1996; 178(2):537–41.

22. Mangwani N, Dash HR, Chauhan A, et al. Bacterial quorum sensing: functional features and potential applications in biotechnology. J Mol Microbiol Biotechnol 2012;22(4):215–27.

23. McDougald D, Rice SA, Barraud N, et al. Should we stay or should we go: mechanisms and ecological consequences for biofilm dispersal. Nat Rev Microbiol 2011;10(1):39–50.

24. Valentini M, Filloux A. Biofilms and cyclic di-GMP (c-di-GMP) signaling: lessons from *Pseudomonas aeruginosa* and other bacteria. J Biol Chem 2016;291(24): 12547–55.

25. Karatan E, Watnick P. Signals, regulatory networks, and materials that build and break bacterial biofilms. Microbiol Mol Biol Rev 2009;73(2):310–47.

26. Olsen I. Biofilm-specific antibiotic tolerance and resistance. Eur J Clin Microbiol Infect Dis 2015;34(5):877–86.

27. Lebeaux D, Ghigo JM, Beloin C. Biofilm-related infections: bridging the gap between clinical management and fundamental aspects of recalcitrance toward antibiotics. Microbiol Mol Biol Rev 2014;78(3):510–43.

28. Conlon BP, Rowe SE, Lewis K. Persister cells in biofilm associated infections. Adv Exp Med Biol 2015;831:1–9.

29. Thuptimdang P, Limpiyakorn T, McEvoy J, et al. Effect of silver nanoparticles on *Pseudomonas putida* biofilms at different stages of maturity. J Hazard Mater 2015;290:127–33.

30. Hausner M, Wuertz S. High rates of conjugation in bacterial biofilms as determined by quantitative in situ analysis. Appl Environ Microbiol 1999;65(8):3710–3.

31. Ryder VJ, Chopra I, O'Neill AJ. Increased mutability of staphylococci in biofilms as a consequence of oxidative stress. PLoS One 2012;7(10):e47695.

32. Krol JE, Wojtowicz AJ, Rogers LM, et al. Invasion of *E. coli* biofilms by antibiotic resistance plasmids. Plasmid 2013;70(1):110–9.

33. Safdar N, Fine JP, Maki DG. Meta-analysis: methods for diagnosing intravascular device-related bloodstream infection. Ann Intern Med 2005;142(6):451–66.

34. Mermel LA, Allon M, Bouza E, et al. Clinical practice guidelines for the diagnosis and management of intravascular catheter-related infection: 2009 Update by the Infectious Diseases Society of America. Clin Infect Dis 2009;49(1):1–45.

35. Raad I, Hanna HA, Alakech B, et al. Differential time to positivity: a useful method for diagnosing catheter-related bloodstream infections. Ann Intern Med 2004;140(1):18–25.

36. Lindsay D, von Holy A. Bacterial biofilms within the clinical setting: what health-care professionals should know. J Hosp Infect 2006;64(4):313–25.

37. Li L, Mendis N, Trigui H, et al. The importance of the viable but non-culturable state in human bacterial pathogens. Front Microbiol 2014;5:258.

38. Zandri G, Pasquaroli S, Vignaroli C, et al. Detection of viable but non-culturable staphylococci in biofilms from central venous catheters negative on standard microbiological assays. Clin Microbiol Infect 2012;18(7):E259–61.

39. Pasquaroli S, Zandri G, Vignaroli C, et al. Antibiotic pressure can induce the viable but non-culturable state in *Staphylococcus aureus* growing in biofilms. J Antimicrob Chemother 2013;68(8):1812–7.

40. Maduka-Ezeh AN, Greenwood-Quaintance KE, Karau MJ, et al. Antimicrobial susceptibility and biofilm formation of *Staphylococcus epidermidis* small colony variants associated with prosthetic joint infection. Diagn Microbiol Infect Dis 2012;74(3):224–9.

41. Tuchscherr L, Heitmann V, Hussain M, et al. *Staphylococcus aureus* small-colony variants are adapted phenotypes for intracellular persistence. J Infect Dis 2010;202(7):1031–40.

42. Perez K, Patel R. *Staphylococcus epidermidis* small-colony variants are induced by low pH and their frequency reduced by lysosomal alkalinization. J Infect Dis 2017;215(3):488–90.

43. Trampuz A, Piper KE, Jacobson MJ, et al. Sonication of removed hip and knee prostheses for diagnosis of infection. N Engl J Med 2007;357(7):654–63.

44. Erb S, Frei R, Schregenberger K, et al. Sonication for diagnosis of catheter-related infection is not better than traditional roll-plate culture: a prospective cohort study with 975 central venous catheters. Clin Infect Dis 2014;59(4):541–4.

45. Bereza PL, Ekiel A, Augusciak-Duma A, et al. Identification of silent prosthetic joint infection: preliminary report of a prospective controlled study. Int Orthop 2013;37(10):2037–43.

46. Gomez E, Cazanave C, Cunningham SA, et al. Prosthetic joint infection diagnosis using broad-range PCR of biofilms dislodged from knee and hip arthroplasty surfaces using sonication. J Clin Microbiol 2012;50(11):3501–8.

47. Larsen MK, Thomsen TR, Moser C, et al. Use of cultivation-dependent and -independent techniques to assess contamination of central venous catheters: a pilot study. BMC Clin Pathol 2008;8:10.
48. Hall-Stoodley L, Hu FZ, Gieseke A, et al. Direct detection of bacterial biofilms on the middle-ear mucosa of children with chronic otitis media. JAMA 2006;296(2): 202–11.
49. Liesman RM, Pritt BS, Maleszewski JJ, et al. Laboratory diagnosis of infective endocarditis. J Clin Microbiol 2017;55(9):2599–608.
50. Tunney MM, Patrick S, Gorman SP, et al. Improved detection of infection in hip replacements. A currently underestimated problem. J Bone Joint Surg Br 1998; 80(4):568–72.
51. Costerton JW, Post JC, Ehrlich GD, et al. New methods for the detection of orthopedic and other biofilm infections. FEMS Immunol Med Microbiol 2011; 61(2):133–40.
52. Stoodley P, Conti SF, DeMeo PJ, et al. Characterization of a mixed MRSA/MRSE biofilm in an explanted total ankle arthroplasty. FEMS Immunol Med Microbiol 2011;62(1):66–74.
53. De Vecchi E, Bottagisio M, Bortolin M, et al. Improving the bacterial recovery by using dithiothreitol with aerobic and anaerobic broth in biofilm-related prosthetic and joint infections. Adv Exp Med Biol 2017;973:31–9.
54. Parry JA, Karau MJ, Kakar S, et al. Disclosing agents for the intraoperative identification of biofilms on orthopedic implants. J Arthroplasty 2017;32(8):2501–4.
55. Stoodley P, Nistico L, Johnson S, et al. Direct demonstration of viable *Staphylococcus aureus* biofilms in an infected total joint arthroplasty. A case report. J Bone Joint Surg Am 2008;90(8):1751–8.
56. Walker JT, Verran J, Boyd RD, et al. Microscopy methods to investigate structure of potable water biofilms. Methods Enzymol 2001;337:243–55.
57. O'Grady NP, Alexander M, Burns LA, et al. Guidelines for the prevention of intravascular catheter-related infections. Clin Infect Dis 2011;52(9):e162–93.
58. Swartjes JJ, Sharma PK, van Kooten TG, et al. Current developments in antimicrobial surface coatings for biomedical applications. Curr Med Chem 2015; 22(18):2116–29.
59. Darouiche RO, Raad II, Heard SO, et al. A comparison of two antimicrobial-impregnated central venous catheters. Catheter Study Group. N Engl J Med 1999;340(1):1–8.
60. Marciante KD, Veenstra DL, Lipsky BA, et al. Which antimicrobial impregnated central venous catheter should we use? Modeling the costs and outcomes of antimicrobial catheter use. Am J Infect Control 2003;31(1):1–8.
61. Rupp ME, Lisco SJ, Lipsett PA, et al. Effect of a second-generation venous catheter impregnated with chlorhexidine and silver sulfadiazine on central catheter-related infections: a randomized, controlled trial. Ann Intern Med 2005;143(8): 570–80.
62. Marschall J, Lane MA, Beekmann SE, et al. Current management of prosthetic joint infections in adults: results of an Emerging Infections Network survey. Int J Antimicrob Agents 2013;41(3):272–7.
63. Kollef MH, Afessa B, Anzueto A, et al. Silver-coated endotracheal tubes and incidence of ventilator-associated pneumonia: the NASCENT randomized trial. JAMA 2008;300(7):805–13.
64. Fabbri S, Johnston DA, Rmaile A, et al. *Streptococcus mutans* biofilm transient viscoelastic fluid behaviour during high-velocity microsprays. J Mech Behav Biomed Mater 2016;59:197–206.

65. Berra L, Coppadoro A, Bittner EA, et al. A clinical assessment of the Mucus Shaver: a device to keep the endotracheal tube free from secretions. Crit Care Med 2012;40(1):119–24.

66. Del Pozo JL, Rouse MS, Euba G, et al. Prevention of *Staphylococcus epidermidis* biofilm formation using electrical current. J Appl Biomater Funct Mater 2014; 12(2):81–3.

67. Vergidis P, Rouse MS, Euba G, et al. Treatment with linezolid or vancomycin in combination with rifampin is effective in an animal model of methicillin-resistant *Staphylococcus aureus* foreign body osteomyelitis. Antimicrob Agents Chemother 2011;55(3):1182–6.

68. Abdi-Ali A, Mohammadi-Mehr M, Agha Alaei Y. Bactericidal activity of various antibiotics against biofilm-producing *Pseudomonas aeruginosa*. Int J Antimicrob Agents 2006;27(3):196–200.

69. Curtin J, Cormican M, Fleming G, et al. Linezolid compared with eperezolid, vancomycin, and gentamicin in an in vitro model of antimicrobial lock therapy for *Staphylococcus epidermidis* central venous catheter-related biofilm infections. Antimicrob Agents Chemother 2003;47(10):3145–8.

70. Vergidis P, Schmidt-Malan SM, Mandrekar JN, et al. Comparative activities of vancomycin, tigecycline and rifampin in a rat model of methicillin-resistant *Staphylococcus aureus* osteomyelitis. J Infect 2015;70(6):609–15.

71. John AK, Baldoni D, Haschke M, et al. Efficacy of daptomycin in implant-associated infection due to methicillin-resistant *Staphylococcus aureus*: importance of combination with rifampin. Antimicrob Agents Chemother 2009;53(7): 2719–24.

72. Mihailescu R, Furustrand Tafin U, Corvec S, et al. High activity of Fosfomycin and Rifampin against methicillin-resistant *Staphylococcus aureus* biofilm in vitro and in an experimental foreign-body infection model. Antimicrob Agents Chemother 2014;58(5):2547–53.

73. Park KH, Greenwood-Quaintance KE, Mandrekar J, et al. Activity of tedizolid in methicillin-resistant *Staphylococcus aureus* experimental foreign body-associated osteomyelitis. Antimicrob Agents Chemother 2016;60(11):6568–72.

74. Fernandez J, Greenwood-Quaintance KE, Patel R. in vitro activity of dalbavancin against biofilms of staphylococci isolated from prosthetic joint infections. Diagn Microbiol Infect Dis 2016;85(4):449–51.

75. Neudorfer K, Schmidt-Malan SM, Patel R. Dalbavancin is active *in vitro* against biofilms formed by dalbavancin-susceptible enterococci. Diagn Microbiol Infect Dis 2018;90(1):58–63.

76. Yan Q, Karau MJ, Patel R. *In vitro* activity of oritavancin against biofilms of staphylococci isolated from prosthetic joint infection. Abstract presented at ASM Microbe. Diagn Microbiol Infect Dis 2018. [Epub ahead of print].

77. Monzon M, Oteiza C, Leiva J, et al. Biofilm testing of *Staphylococcus epidermidis* clinical isolates: low performance of vancomycin in relation to other antibiotics. Diagn Microbiol Infect Dis 2002;44(4):319–24.

78. Budhani RK, Struthers JK. Interaction of *Streptococcus pneumoniae* and *Moraxella catarrhalis*: investigation of the indirect pathogenic role of beta-lactamase-producing moraxellae by use of a continuous-culture biofilm system. Antimicrob Agents Chemother 1998;42(10):2521–6.

79. Adam B, Baillie GS, Douglas LJ. Mixed species biofilms of *Candida albicans* and *Staphylococcus epidermidis*. J Med Microbiol 2002;51(4):344–9.

80. Sanders J, Pithie A, Ganly P, et al. A prospective double-blind randomized trial comparing intraluminal ethanol with heparinized saline for the prevention of

catheter-associated bloodstream infection in immunosuppressed haematology patients. J Antimicrob Chemother 2008;62(4):809 15.

81. Yahav D, Rozen-Zvi B, Gafter-Gvili A, et al. Antimicrobial lock solutions for the prevention of infections associated with intravascular catheters in patients undergoing hemodialysis: systematic review and meta-analysis of randomized, controlled trials. Clin Infect Dis 2008;47(1):83–93.

82. Fortun J, Grill F, Martin-Davila P, et al. Treatment of long-term intravascular catheter-related bacteraemia with antibiotic-lock therapy. J Antimicrob Chemother 2006;58(4):816–21.

83. May RM, Magin CM, Mann EE, et al. An engineered micropattern to reduce bacterial colonization, platelet adhesion and fibrin sheath formation for improved biocompatibility of central venous catheters. Clin Transl Med 2015;4:9.

84. Donlan RM. Preventing biofilms of clinically relevant organisms using bacteriophage. Trends Microbiol 2009;17(2):66–72.

85. Curtin JJ, Donlan RM. Using bacteriophages to reduce formation of catheter-associated biofilms by Staphylococcus epidermidis. Antimicrob Agents Chemother 2006;50(4):1268–75.

86. Fu W, Forster T, Mayer O, et al. Bacteriophage cocktail for the prevention of biofilm formation by *Pseudomonas aeruginosa* on catheters in an in vitro model system. Antimicrob Agents Chemother 2010;54(1):397–404.

87. Akanda ZZ, Taha M, Abdelbary H. Current review - the rise of bacteriophage as a unique therapeutic platform in treating peri-prosthetic joint infections. J Orthop Res 2018;36(4):1051–60.

88. Kaplan JB. Biofilm matrix-degrading enzymes. Methods Mol Biol 2014;1147:203–13.

89. Okshevsky M, Regina VR, Meyer RL. Extracellular DNA as a target for biofilm control. Curr Opin Biotechnol 2015;33:73–80.

90. Darouiche RO, Mansouri MD, Gawande PV, et al. Antimicrobial and antibiofilm efficacy of triclosan and dispersin B combination. J Antimicrob Chemother 2009;64(1):88–93.

91. Schuch R, Khan BK, Raz A, et al. Bacteriophage lysin CF-301, a potent antistaphylococcal biofilm agent. Antimicrob Agents Chemother 2017;61(7) [pii: e02666-16].

92. Nett JE, Cabezas-Olcoz J, Marchillo K, et al. Targeting fibronectin to disrupt *in vivo Candida albicans* biofilms. Antimicrob Agents Chemother 2016;60(5):3152–5.

93. Spaulding CN, Klein RD, Ruer S, et al. Selective depletion of uropathogenic *E. coli* from the gut by a FimH antagonist. Nature 2017;546(7659):528–32.

94. Totsika M, Kostakioti M, Hannan TJ, et al. A FimH inhibitor prevents acute bladder infection and treats chronic cystitis caused by multidrug-resistant uropathogenic *Escherichia coli* ST131. J Infect Dis 2013;208(6):921–8.

95. Bjarnsholt T, Givskov M. Quorum sensing inhibitory drugs as next generation antimicrobials: worth the effort? Curr Infect Dis Rep 2008;10(1):22–8.

96. Sultana ST, Call DR, Beyenal H. Eradication of *Pseudomonas aeruginosa* biofilms and persister cells using an electrochemical scaffold and enhanced antibiotic susceptibility. NPJ Biofilms Microbiomes 2016;2:2.

97. Gallo J, Panacek A, Prucek R, et al. Silver nanocoating technology in the prevention of prosthetic joint infection. Materials (Basel) 2016;9(5) [pii:E337].

98. Schutz CA, Juillerat-Jeanneret L, Mueller H, et al. Therapeutic nanoparticles in clinics and under clinical evaluation. Nanomedicine (Lond) 2013;8(3):449–67.

99. Wang LS, Gupta A, Rotello VM. Nanomaterials for the treatment of bacterial biofilms. ACS Infect Dis 2016;2(1):3–4.
100. Duncan B, Li X, Landis RF, et al. Nanoparticle-stabilized capsules for the treatment of bacterial biofilms. ACS Nano 2015;9(8):7775–82.
101. Giri K, Yepes LR, Duncan B, et al. Targeting bacterial biofilms via surface engineering of gold nanoparticles. RSC Adv 2015;5(128):105551–9.
102. Forier K, Raemdonck K, De Smedt SC, et al. Lipid and polymer nanoparticles for drug delivery to bacterial biofilms. J Control Release 2014;190:607–23.
103. Rukavina Z, Vanic Z. Current trends in development of liposomes for targeting bacterial biofilms. Pharmaceutics 2016;8(2) [pii:E18].
104. Machado MC, Tarquinio KM, Webster TJ. Decreased *Staphylococcus aureus* biofilm formation on nanomodified endotracheal tubes: a dynamic airway model. Int J Nanomedicine 2012;7:3741–50.
105. Machado MC, Webster TJ. Decreased *Pseudomonas aeruginosa* biofilm formation on nanomodified endotracheal tubes: a dynamic lung model. Int J Nanomedicine 2016;11:3825–31.
106. Schmidt-Malan SM, Karau MJ, Cede J, et al. Antibiofilm activity of low-amperage continuous and intermittent direct electrical current. Antimicrob Agents Chemother 2015;59(8):4610–5.
107. Ruiz-Ruigomez M, Badiola J, Schmidt-Malan SM, et al. Direct electrical current reduces bacterial and yeast biofilm formation. Int J Bacteriol 2016;2016: 9727810.
108. Brinkman CL, Schmidt-Malan SM, Karau MJ, et al. Exposure of bacterial biofilms to electrical current leads to cell death mediated in part by reactive oxygen species. PLoS One 2016;11(12):e0168595.
109. Del Pozo JL, Rouse MS, Euba G, et al. The electricidal effect is active in an experimental model of *Staphylococcus epidermidis* chronic foreign body osteomyelitis. Antimicrob Agents Chemother 2009;53(10):4064–8.
110. Schmidt-Malan SM, Brinkman CL, Greenwood-Quaintance KE, et al. Activity of electrical current in experimental *Propionibacterium acnes* foreign-body osteomyelitis. Antimicrob Agents Chemother 2017;61(2) [pii:e01863-16].
111. Voegele P, Badiola J, Schmidt-Malan SM, et al. Antibiofilm activity of electrical current in a catheter Model. Antimicrob Agents Chemother 2015;60(3):1476–80.
112. del Pozo JL, Rouse MS, Mandrekar JN, et al. The electricidal effect: reduction of *Staphylococcus* and *Pseudomonas* biofilms by prolonged exposure to low-intensity electrical current. Antimicrob Agents Chemother 2009;53(1):41–5.
113. del Pozo JL, Rouse MS, Mandrekar JN, et al. Effect of electrical current on the activities of antimicrobial agents against *Pseudomonas aeruginosa, Staphylococcus aureus*, and *Staphylococcus epidermidis biofilms*. Antimicrob Agents Chemother 2009;53(1):35–40.
114. Sultana ST, Atci E, Babauta JT, et al. Electrochemical scaffold generates localized, low concentration of hydrogen peroxide that inhibits bacterial pathogens and biofilms. Sci Rep 2015;5:14908.

UNITED STATES POSTAL SERVICE ®

Statement of Ownership, Management, and Circulation
(All Periodicals Publications Except Requester Publications)

1. Publication Title	2. Publication Number	3. Filing Date
INFECTIOUS DISEASE CLINICS OF NORTH AMERICA	001 – 556	9/18/2018

4. Issue Frequency	5. Number of Issues Published Annually	6. Annual Subscription Price
MAR, JUN, SEP, DEC	4	$319.00

7. Complete Mailing Address of Known Office of Publication (Not printer) (Street, city, county, state, and ZIP+4®)

ELSEVIER INC.
230 Park Avenue, Suite 800
New York, NY 10169

Contact Person
STEPHEN R. BUSHING

Telephone (Include area code)
215-239-3688

8. Complete Mailing Address of Headquarters or General Business Office of Publisher (Not printer)

ELSEVIER INC.
230 Park Avenue, Suite 800
New York, NY 10169

9. Full Names and Complete Mailing Addresses of Publisher, Editor, and Managing Editor (Do not leave blank)

Publisher (Name and complete mailing address)

TAYLOR E BALL, ELSEVIER INC.
1600 JOHN F KENNEDY BLVD. SUITE 1800
PHILADELPHIA, PA 19103-2899

Editor (Name and complete mailing address)

KERRY HOLLAND, ELSEVIER INC.
1600 JOHN F KENNEDY BLVD. SUITE 1800
PHILADELPHIA, PA 19103-2899

Managing Editor (Name and complete mailing address)

PATRICK MANLEY, ELSEVIER INC.
1600 JOHN F KENNEDY BLVD. SUITE 1800
PHILADELPHIA, PA 19103-2899

10. Owner (Do not leave blank. If the publication is owned by a corporation, give the name and address of the corporation immediately followed by the names and addresses of all stockholders owning or holding 1 percent or more of the total amount of stock. If not owned by a corporation, give the names and addresses of the individual owners. If owned by a partnership or other unincorporated firm, give its name and address as well as those of each individual owner. If the publication is published by a nonprofit organization, give its name and address.)

Full Name	Complete Mailing Address
WHOLLY OWNED SUBSIDIARY OF REED/ELSEVIER, US HOLDINGS	1600 JOHN F KENNEDY BLVD. SUITE 1800 PHILADELPHIA, PA 19103-2899

11. Known Bondholders, Mortgagees, and Other Security Holders Owning or Holding 1 Percent or More of Total Amount of Bonds, Mortgages, or Other Securities. If none, check box ▶ ☐ None

Full Name	Complete Mailing Address
N/A	

12. Tax Status (For completion by nonprofit organizations authorized to mail at nonprofit rates) (Check one)
The purpose, function, and nonprofit status of this organization and the exempt status for federal income tax purposes:
☒ Has Not Changed During Preceding 12 Months
☐ Has Changed During Preceding 12 Months (Publisher must submit explanation of change with this statement)

PS Form 3526, July 2014 [Page 1 of 4 (see instructions page 4)] PSN: 7530-01-000-9931 PRIVACY NOTICE: See our privacy policy on www.usps.com

---

13. Publication Title	14. Issue Date for Circulation Data Below
INFECTIOUS DISEASE CLINICS OF NORTH AMERICA	JUNE 2018

15. Extent and Nature of Circulation		Average No. Copies Each Issue During Preceding 12 Months	No. Copies of Single Issue Published Nearest to Filing Date
a. Total Number of Copies (Net press run)		255	328
b. Paid Circulation (By Mail and Outside the Mail)	(1) Mailed Outside-County Paid Subscriptions Stated on PS Form 3541 (Include paid distribution above nominal rate, advertiser's proof copies, and exchange copies)	151	184
	(2) Mailed In-County Paid Subscriptions Stated on PS Form 3541 (Include paid distribution above nominal rate, advertiser's proof copies, and exchange copies)	0	0
	(3) Paid Distribution Outside the Mails Including Sales Through Dealers and Carriers, Street Vendors, Counter Sales, and Other Paid Distribution Outside USPS®	48	61
	(4) Paid Distribution by Other Classes of Mail Through the USPS (e.g., First-Class Mail®)	0	0
c. Total Paid Distribution (Sum of 15b (1), (2), (3), and (4))		199	245
d. Free or Nominal Rate Distribution (By Mail and Outside the Mail)	(1) Free or Nominal Rate Outside-County Copies included on PS Form 3541	44	68
	(2) Free or Nominal Rate In-County Copies Included on PS Form 3541	0	0
	(3) Free or Nominal Rate Copies Mailed at Other Classes Through the USPS (e.g. First-Class Mail)	0	0
	(4) Free or Nominal Rate Distribution Outside the Mail (Carriers or other means)	0	0
e. Total Free or Nominal Rate Distribution (Sum of 15d (1), (2), (3) and (4))		44	68
f. Total Distribution (Sum of 15c and 15e)		243	313
g. Copies not Distributed (See Instructions to Publishers #4 (page #3))		12	15
h. Total (Sum of 15f and g)		255	328
i. Percent Paid (15c divided by 15f times 100)		81.89%	78.27%

* If you are claiming electronic copies, go to line 16 on page 3. If you are not claiming electronic copies, skip to line 17 on page 3.

16. Electronic Copy Circulation	Average No. Copies Each Issue During Preceding 12 Months	No. Copies of Single Issue Published Nearest to Filing Date
a. Paid Electronic Copies	0	0
b. Total Paid Print Copies (Line 15c) + Paid Electronic Copies (Line 16a)	199	245
c. Total Print Distribution (Line 15f) + Paid Electronic Copies (Line 16a)	243	313
d. Percent Paid (Both Print & Electronic Copies) (16b divided by 16c × 100)	81.89%	78.27%

☒ I certify that 50% of all my distributed copies (electronic and print) are paid above a nominal price.

17. Publication of Statement of Ownership

☒ If the publication is a general publication, publication of this statement is required. Will be printed in the DECEMBER 2018 issue of this publication. ☐ Publication not required.

18. Signature and Title of Editor, Publisher, Business Manager, or Owner

STEPHEN R. BUSHING – INVENTORY DISTRIBUTION CONTROL MANAGER

[signature] Stephen R. Bushing

Date 9/18/2018

I certify that all information furnished on this form is true and complete. I understand that anyone who furnishes false or misleading information on this form or who omits material or information requested on the form may be subject to criminal sanctions (including fines and imprisonment) and/or civil sanctions (including civil penalties).

PS Form 3526, July 2014 (Page 2 of 4) PRIVACY NOTICE: See our privacy policy on www.usps.com

Moving?

Make sure your subscription moves with you!

To notify us of your new address, find your **Clinics Account Number** (located on your mailing label above your name), and contact customer service at:

Email: journalscustomerservice-usa@elsevier.com

800-654-2452 (subscribers in the U.S. & Canada)
314-447-8871 (subscribers outside of the U.S. & Canada)

Fax number: 314-447-8029

Elsevier Health Sciences Division
Subscription Customer Service
3251 Riverport Lane
Maryland Heights, MO 63043

*To ensure uninterrupted delivery of your subscription, please notify us at least 4 weeks in advance of move.

Printed and bound by CPI Group (UK) Ltd, Croydon, CR0 4YY

08/05/2025

01864737-0003